D1326867

Radiographic Imaging

For Churchill Livingstone:

Senior Commissioning Editor: Sarena Wolfaard
Project Development Manager: Dinah Thom
Project Manager: Andrea Hill
Design Direction: Judith Wright

Radiographic Imaging

A Practical Approach

Chris Gunn MA TDCR
CG Training, Retford, Nottinghamshire, UK

THIRD EDITION

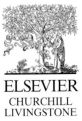

ELSEVIER
CHURCHILL
LIVINGSTONE
EDINBURGH LONDON NEW YORK OXFORD PHILADELPHIA ST LOUIS SYDNEY TORONTO 2002

CHURCHILL LIVINGSTONE
An imprint of Elsevier Limited

First edition 1988
Second edition 1994
Third edition 2002
   Reprinted 2005 (twice)

ISBN 0 443 07115 2

British Library Cataloguing in Publication Data
A catalogue record for this book is available from the British Library

Library of Congress Cataloguing in Publication Data
A catalogue record for this book is available from the Library of Congress

Note
Medical knowledge is constantly changing. As new information becomes
available, changes in treatment, procedures, equipment and the use of drugs
become necessary. The author, contributor and the publishers have, as far as it
is possible, taken care to ensure that the information given in this text is
accurate and up to date. However, readers are strongly advised to confirm
that the information, especially with regard to drug usage, complies with the
latest legislation and standards of practice.

                                                            The Publisher

 your source for books,
journals and multimedia
in the health sciences
www.elsevierhealth.com

Working together to grow
libraries in developing countries

www.elsevier.com | www.bookaid.org | www.sabre.org

ELSEVIER   BOOK AID International   Sabre Foundation

The
publisher's
policy is to use
paper manufactured
from sustainable forests

Printed in China

Contents

Preface to the Third Edition

A number of years have passed since the second edition of this book appeared. Since then, computers have become commonplace in imaging departments, and advances with regard to picture archiving and communication systems (PACS), the advent of the Digital Imaging and Communication in Medicine project (DICOM) and the introduction of image analysis have meant that their future is assured. In spite of that, many departments still use conventional films and cassettes and therefore I have retained these more traditional aspects of radiographic imaging.

European law now has a greater impact on imaging departments and, with the current emphasis on environmental concerns, more legislation is appearing aimed at regulating the reduction and safe disposal of waste products. The information supplied with chemicals and the personal and environmental issues surrounding them are also gaining attention; Section 4, on environmental considerations and legislation, has therefore been expanded to give an indication of the type of information that is being provided. I have also, more generally, introduced a number of additional headings and lists into the text in order to make the information more easily accessible.

The pace of change is such that virtually no textbook is able to keep up with the advances in technology. Fortunately much of the information is now available on the internet and for that reason I have included details of some useful websites together with the more traditional references. These sites are kept up to date by the manufacturers and provide a valuable source of additional information on new products.

Derrick Roberts and Nigel Smith were the original authors of *Radiographic Imaging*, and I was privileged to listen to both of them lecture on the practical aspects of photography. Their extensive knowledge of the subject provided a sound basis for this book and their hard work must be acknowledged as they provided the foundation for this present edition.

Finally, I would like to thank the many manufacturers who sent me literature and those who keep their very comprehensive websites up to date. It is very clear that we could no longer manage without computers – the information they provide and their ability to transfer information throughout the health community are something that can only be of benefit to patients.

Retford 2002   C. Gunn

Preface to the First Edition

It is often argued that radiography is more art than science. Whilst the argument has never been settled, it is indisputable that a great deal of radiography requires a practical approach.

This book has been written to satisfy the need for more practical knowledge in the imaging sciences. To this end every chapter, wherever possible, connects the theory with the practice.

The book is aimed at students in the field of diagnostic imaging, from graduate and post-graduate radiographic students to trainee radiologists. The book can be of use as a reference within the imaging department and as a manual of photographic quality assurance and fault finding which is easy to understand and read.

Particular attention has been paid to the subject areas where our experience has indicated most of the common misconceptions occur. The science of imaging is too complex a subject to be covered by one book. If further information is required in specialised areas, the reader is referred to other experts in the field.

It should be added that the interpretations expressed in this book are our own and may conflict with the long-standing opinions of others.

D. P. Roberts
N. L. Smith

Chapter 1
Monitor photography

CHAPTER CONTENTS

INTRODUCTION

Monitor photography is the filming of images from a cathode ray tube (CRT). From its infancy in the early 1970s, it has grown to become a major part of diagnostic imaging departments. Initially, monitor photography was associated with the early CT imaging systems where a simple camera was bolted onto the diagnostic monitor, and films were then made of the images on the monitor. These cameras took one exposure at a time, usually on 5×4 in film.

There are now video imagers available which contain their own monitor and camera and are totally dedicated to monitor photography. These imagers can produce as many as 25 exposures on one film and are known as multiformat cameras.

With the advent of ultrasound, computed tomography, digital radiography, MRI and other technologies, where the only image available is displayed on a monitor, a dedicated video imager is now a necessity and high resolution imaging is essential. Hard copy images, either on paper or on film, are required. The patient's notes carry a paper copy of the image and the original film is used either as a 'master' in the filing system, or for higher quality imaging.

These new technologies have created demands for film (and paper) capable of recording high quality images, and which responds to the phosphors used in the imagers. The purpose of this chapter is to discuss briefly the way the image is produced on the monitor itself and to consider the way the film is designed to cope with the stringent demands placed upon it.

THE CHARACTERISTICS OF THE VIDEO IMAGE

The following descriptions relate to the imaging process from the television camera to the monitor. The principles obviously apply equally to the image production on the imaging camera monitor.

Persistence of vision

The moving video image relies on the principle of persistence of vision, the same principle used in cinema photography. To produce a flicker-free, moving image, 25 frames per second are required (see p. 12).

Interlacing

Consider one still picture of one frame. This frame is made up of two fields which consist, in a 625-line system, of 312.5 lines each. The two fields when combined add up to the one complete frame of 625 lines. If you observe the picture very closely you will see that it is made up of minute dots along the horizontal scanning lines. These dots are the resolutions of individual pixels along the line. If the pixel is considered as having depth, it is referred to as a voxel.

The field is constructed by an electron beam scanning the tube phosphor from top left to bottom right in a series of horizontal lines, as illustrated in Figure 1.1. First the odd lines are scanned, then the even lines. In this way the composite (the frame) is completed.

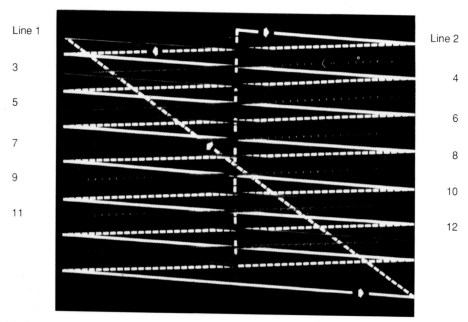

Fig. 1.1 Odd, then even lines are scanned.

This system of constructing the frame is known as 'double interlacing'; it requires sophisticated electronic circuitry to achieve the accurate spacing of the lines which is imperative for high quality images.

The interlacing can be carried still further. For example, × 4 and × 8 interlacing are not uncommon and will produce images which, to all intents and purposes, are line free (Fig. 1.2).

Image display

The display system used in most imaging departments is referred to as a monitor. This bears a strong family resemblance to a television set, but there is a main intrinsic difference between the two, apart from the fact that a diagnostic system is usually a closed system (i.e. the images arrive by wire, rather than by an aerial):

In a *television set*:

- The video signal arrives at the tube through various electronics and radio frequency (RF) circuitry.

In a *monitor*:

- The video signal is fed directly to the processing circuitry without interference.

On some *colour monitors*:

- An RGB input is often available (this input accepts directly the red, green and blue signals offered by the colour video signal).

THE TELEVISION CAMERA

Two of the most common cameras are the Videcon and Plumbicon cameras. The image is formed in a similar way to the monitor image but the electrons generated have to scan the signal plate of the tube and gain information about the amount of light and dark areas formed on the signal plate. The plate is scanned in a similar way to the monitor, in regular horizontal lines. The video signal is generated in pulses which correspond to the image formed on the signal plate. This signal is formed by (in the Videcon) tiny globules embedded in the signal plate, discharging like condensers.

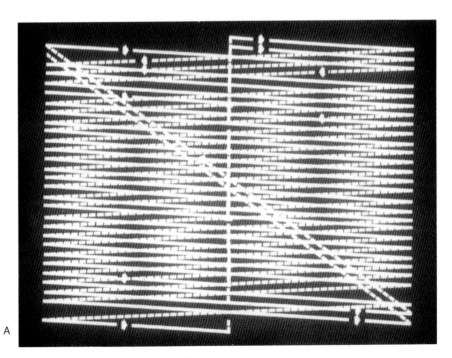

A

Fig. 1.2 Multiple interlacing: (A) × 2 interlacing. (*Figure continues*)

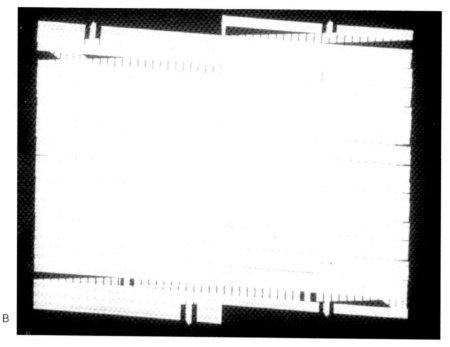

B

Fig. 1.2 (*continued*) Multiple interlacing: (B) raster lines almost disappear.

BANDWIDTH AND RESOLUTION

The *bandwidth* of a system is defined as follows:

> **The bandwidth is the difference between the maximum and minimum frequency that the system has to cope with.**

In a 625-line system, a *horizontal* resolution of 300 lines, which approaches equal horizontal and vertical resolution, is a fairly good system (Fig. 1.3).

The maximum frequency can then be calculated by multiplying the maximum number of cycles (300) by the number of scan lines per frame and the number of frames per second, i.e.:

$$\underset{\text{cycles}}{300} \times \underset{\text{lines}}{625} \times \underset{\text{frames}}{25} = 4\ 687\ 500$$

A *maximum* frequency of almost 5 million hertz is required, i.e. 5 MHz.

The minimum frequency required will be when only one cycle is to be resolved, i.e. when the screen is half black, half white – a highly unlikely occurrence but a good theoretical concept (Fig. 1.4). In this case the calculation is:

$$1 \times 625 \times 25 = 15\ 625$$

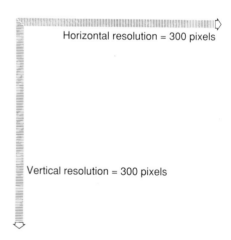

Horizontal resolution = 300 pixels

Vertical resolution = 300 pixels

Fig. 1.3 A monitor which could offer equal horizontal and vertical resolution would produce reasonable resolution.

This figure represents the *minimum* frequency to be dealt with.

Therefore, the bandwidth required to cope with the maximum and minimum frequencies is:

$$4\ 687\ 500 - 15\ 625 = 4\ 671\ 875$$

or, 4.67 MHz.

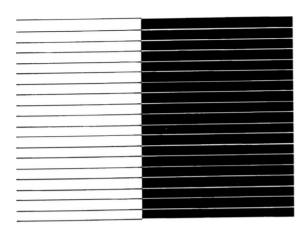

Fig. 1.4 The simplest possible signal would be half the screen white and half black.

This figure is for an uncomplicated black and white image. For a coloured image the figure for bandwidth would be much greater. Brightness and colour levels, which increase the demands for bandwidth, would also have to be taken into account.

PHOSPHORS

There are a number of phosphors commonly in use as the coating for the monitor tube. They each have a characteristic light emission when stimulated by the electron beam. The most common are listed below:

P45 'White' (a mixture of blue and green)
P11 Blue
P31 ⎱
P24 ⎰ Both green-emitting phosphors
P4 ⎱
P40 ⎰ Both 'white' phosphors, i.e. blue and green

THE IMAGING CAMERA

Imaging cameras were initially simple 'bolt on' cameras linked to a conventional monitor, sometimes even to the diagnostic monitor.

The film was usually carried in a dark slide cassette, usually double-sided. The film was loaded into both sides of the cassette with the emulsion side facing outwards. To expose the emulsion, a slide was removed when the cassette was in the camera. After exposure, the film was covered with the slide and the process was repeated for the second film.

When the matrix size of the diagnostic equipment was small, very few demands were put on the imaging camera; but matrices began to increase in size until it was realised that the definition required was outstripping the performance of simple cameras and monitors. From this point onwards the dedicated imaging camera was inevitable.

The evolution of the imaging camera

Figure 1.5 shows the development of the imaging camera, from the simple 'bolt on' to the multiformat camera of today.

Cameras have evolved from utilising a simple, usually curved-screen monitor to microprocessor-controlled dedicated cameras.

The second type of camera consisted of a monitor with a flat screen, using only one size of film and giving only one specific format. For example, this could be one image on a 18×24 cm film, or four images on a 18×24 cm film. This type of camera then developed into a multiformat camera, where different numbers of images could be stored on the same 18×24 cm film. On some types of these cameras there is also the possibility of using different sizes of film (e.g. a 18×24 cm and a 35×43 cm film). The line diagrams in Figure 1.5 demonstrate the basic principles of operation of the imagers.

Cameras are now 'multiformat, multisized', with microprocessor control and an inbuilt processing machine. These cameras allow a single 35×43 cm film (for example) to image a variety of images from different format sizes. Modern cameras are constrained by certain parameters.

Parameters

The parameters for an imaging camera can be laid down as follows:

1. Type of monitor
2. Stability

A Bolted directly to diagnostic monitor

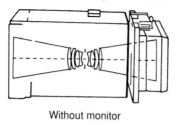

Without monitor

B Integrated monitor

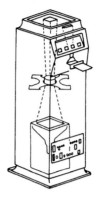

C With monitor plus automatic film transport and processing

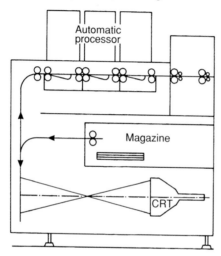

Fig. 1.5 Development of the imaging camera.

3. Exposure
4. Interlacing
5. The optical system.

Each of these will be discussed in turn. These parameters apply equally to a single format or a multiformat camera.

Type of imaging monitor

The monitor must be flat faced, to avoid edge distortion of the image. The phosphors most frequently used in monitors are listed on page 5.

Stability

The raster pattern should be extremely stable, to avoid any loss of resolution of the image. This is sometimes highlighted when changing from a very fast (diffusion transfer, 3000 ISO-type) film, to conventional imaging film. It is sometimes noted that on the slow film the raster lines disappear and this is usually attributed to 'loss of definition'. But with an extremely fast film, perhaps two or three fields are all that are needed to form an image. Even if the raster lines are slightly unstable, they will clearly be seen on only three fields. With a slow film, perhaps 14 fields will be required. Any raster instability will be clearly demonstrated, as the raster lines will be blurred or possibly absent.

Exposure

In Europe the frequency of the mains supply is 50 hertz. This means that there are 50 fields per second produced on the monitor. The *minimum* exposure possible is 0.04 seconds, to give one complete frame. An exposure length must guarantee that at least two fields are imaged; any shorter exposure will result in only a partial frame, perhaps only one field, and therefore only half the information would be imaged.

An improvement on 'time' exposures is to translate the exposure time into the number of fields imaged for each exposure. Users dial the number of fields they wish to image, and the camera – electronically – does the rest.

With a monitor image it is important that brightness is not increased to a point at which unsharpness occurs, due to phosphor flare; therefore exposure length is used to determine blackness rather than increasing the brightness on the cathode ray tube (CRT).

The intensity of light is achieved by the number of electrons hitting a particular spot on the CRT. If the number of electrons is increased (the equivalent of increasing brightness), the spot size at the CRT becomes larger, increasing unsharpness. This effect is demonstrated on a viewing monitor, where sharpness is at its best at the black end of the image and decreases as the image becomes whiter.

Interlacing

The greater the interlacing, the less likelihood there is of raster lines being displayed (see p. 2).

Optical system

Problems associated with the optical system may include:

1. Vignetting – shading round the image
2. Lens imperfections, for example:
   Spherical aberration – a difference in focusing between the edge and the centre
   Chromatic aberration – the non-convergence of the different coloured rays
   Astigmatism – light from a point not focusing to a point
3. Density uniformity – a change in density across the film.

The above factors can be minimised by:

In-line optics. The image, lens and film are aligned and used with a flat screen monitor to overcome most of the distortion problems.

Increasing the size of the CRT. As by using a CRT larger than the image field: for example, using a 17.5 cm monitor with a 12.5 cm imaging field can reduce vignetting.

Electronic manipulation of the density profile. Density uniformity can be a problem, as often there is a fall-off of light to the edge of the film. Therefore the density profile is changed so that the edge brightness on the monitor is higher than the centre brightness.

Using only the centre of the lens system. The centre of the lens is where resolution is at its highest. Therefore by only allowing a choice of high f-stop numbers (i.e. f 8, f 16, etc.), or by offering no choice at all, resolution can be improved. Unlike in conventional photography, the depth of field (associated with low f-stop numbers such as f 2.8 and low resolution) is not important as the 'image' lies on a phosphor which is only microns thick.

Lens manufacture. If the camera is used for coloured images, a higher quality lens will be required to prevent chromatic aberration.

THE IMAGING FILM

The film used for monitor photography has some features which are unique. It is a single-coated film and construction details are given in Chapter 4 (Film materials, p. 59).

As there is a relationship between the phosphor and the type of film, the following features should be considered when selecting a film for use with a specific system:

The emulsion

The characteristics of the emulsion are determined by the phosphor used in coating the monitor. As can be seen from the list above (p. 5), these range from a solely blue-emitting phosphor through to green-emitting phosphors, plus combinations of blue and green.

Clearly a purely monochromatic film would not respond to the green emissions of, for example, a P31 phosphor. If a monochromatic film was used in this situation, a very 'grainy' image would be produced. The 'grain' is the unresolved green emissions which leave blanks in the image. Figure 1.6A shows the spectral sensitivity curve of a typical imaging film, superimposed onto the emissions of P4, P24, P31 and P11 phosphors. A monochromatic film would be unable to respond to the green emission of the phosphor, and indeed contrast changes significantly with the type of phosphor used (Fig. 1.6B).

The choice of emulsion type is therefore orthochromatic.

Emulsion contrast

Film can be of either low contrast or high contrast. Low contrast film should be used for *all* imaging. This is because the raster lines on the monitor image are the highest contrast available on the image, and a high contrast film would merely amplify this high subject contrast.

Historically, imaging film was always high contrast. With the advent of large usage of film in ultrasound, more users began to demand low contrast emulsion. At first, many people felt that this was just a matter of personal preference whereas in fact there is a strict scientific basis for these decisions.

Low contrast film brings an extended latitude. This would seem to mean that the film would cope with fluctuations in the output of the CRT

within the camera, and the fluctuations would have much less effect.

This argument seems to be reasonable, but the decision about type of contrast really depends on what type of image is being displayed. The main difference between CT/MRI images and ultrasound images is the polarity of the image.

A CT/MRI image has a *black* background, hence the original monitor image background is *white*.

An ultrasound image has a *white* background, hence the original monitor image background is *black*.

Anyone who has cleaned an imaging camera, particularly inside, will understand some of the implications of the above statements.

Any dust on the lens or the inside of the camera body, any scratches on the internal paintwork, will cause flare or scattered light inside the camera body. This flare will, in turn, lead to decreased subject contrast. On an already low contrast film the contrast becomes even lower because of lower maximum density and higher base fog. High contrast film will go a long way towards compensating for these losses.

However, a low contrast film is still better for ultrasonographers because the monitor image background is black and this causes significantly less flare and scatter. Ultrasound also demands a

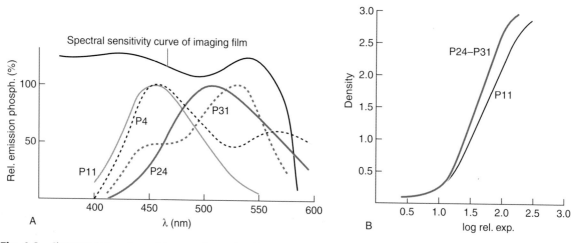

Fig. 1.6 Characteristics of emulsion are determined by the phosphors used in coating the monitor: (A) spectral sensitivity curve of orthochromatic film superimposed onto the emissions of P4, P24, P31 and P11 phosphors; (B) contrast changes significantly depending on type of phosphor used.

long grey scale, particularly in the toe of the curve (see Clear base, p. 53).

To summarise: the general decision, almost worldwide, is that CT/MRI require a high contrast film and ultrasound requires a low contrast film.

SENSITOMETRIC CHARACTERISTICS (*see* Ch. 8, Sensitometry)

In monitor photography it is important not to treat the film in isolation but to remember that it is part of a chain of equipment. It is also important to relate the behaviour of the film to certain changes which take place in the imaging equipment.

Most imagers have three major controls. They are the controls which set *brightness*, *contrast* and *exposure time*. Adjusting any of these controls has a profound effect on the final image quality produced. It is worth considering in some depth what the sensitometric effect is when the controls are adjusted.

Brightness

When the brightness control is adjusted on the monitor, the picture becomes considerably lighter. However, the effect on the film is noted on the log It axis of the characteristic curve. As the brightness goes up (i.e. moves *right* along the log It axis), so the maximum density of the final image moves up the slope of the characteristic curve (Fig. 1.7).

The converse is also true: as brightness is turned down (i.e. moves *left* along the log It axis), the maximum density obtained on the final image goes down.

Contrast

The movement of the contrast control produces a different effect entirely. The function of this adjustment is to alter the brightness range available on the monitor.

Assuming that brightness (and hence maximum density) has already been set, the density *range*

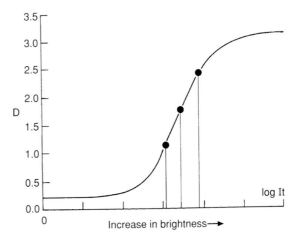

Fig. 1.7   As brightness increases, the maximum density of the final image moves up the slope of the characteristic curve.

obtainable on the final image will be determined by the setting of the contrast control (Fig. 1.8).

Exposure time

If the exposure time is altered, this will have the effect of moving the present brightness range of the subject up or down the log It axis. Short exposures will produce 'thin' images, long exposures will produce dark images.

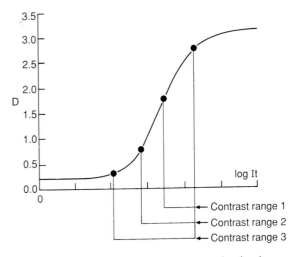

Fig. 1.8   The contrast control determines the density range available on the final image.

Density overall will increase or decrease, but contrast may also increase or decrease if the upper or lower values of the contrast range obtrude into the shoulder or toe of the characteristic curve. In other words, care must be taken to try to keep the parameters of brightness, contrast and exposure time within the region of useful exposure of the characteristic curve of the film (Fig. 1.9).

SIZING OF FILMS

The film sizes for monitor film are many and varied, from conventional sheet film to 75 m roll film.

The list below shows film currently available. (It should be stressed that this list is not comprehensive, but merely illustrative of the formats available.)

Sheet film

9×10 cm
5×4 in
18×24 cm
11×14 in
10×12 in
10×10 cm
5×7 in

8×10 in
14×17 in

Roll film

70 mm $\times$ 45 m
90 mm $\times$ 30 m
105 mm $\times$ 45 m
8 in $\times$ 75 m

It can be seen from the above list that there is a complete pot-pourri of sizes obtainable. Initially, imperial sizing was used (with the 5×4 in size) and then more and more manufacturers entered the field. Metric sizes were then introduced as well, meaning that both imperial and metric sizes are available, a mixture which is now unique in medical imaging.

It will be noted that roll film has been included in the list. Imaging cameras are available to handle such roll film. Instead of handling numerous cassettes in a busy session, the department is able to produce large numbers of images (as many as 1300 on one roll) and then sort them out at a later date.

FILM OR PAPER IMAGES?

Another decision to be made when using an imaging camera is whether to use film or paper for making the hard copy.

A simple example will illustrate the problem. Very often, after returning from holiday, a decision is made to get the slides of the holiday snaps copied and have prints made, so that they can be passed round the family or at work. Anyone who has done this will have experienced the disappointment when they realise that the prints are not as good as the slides. This is not the fault of the paper manufacturer or the laboratory, it is merely the intrinsic difference between the two materials.

A slide image is an image designed to be viewed by *transmitted* light; paper prints are to be viewed by *reflected* light.

Exactly the same rules apply to monitor photography. A film image is designed for transmitted light, a paper image for reflected light. This simple difference accounts for the different behaviour of these two materials.

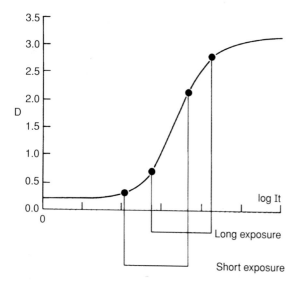

Fig. 1.9 Altering exposure time will shift the preset brightness range up or down the log It axis: short exposures produce 'thin' images, long exposures produce dark images.

Transmitted light image

In Chapter 8 (Sensitometry), percentage transmission is discussed and it is pointed out that at density 2.0 only 1% of the incident light actually reaches the eye. The maximum density reached on film depends largely on the amount of silver that the manufacturer is prepared to put in the film. Figures significantly higher than density 2.0 could be reached quite easily, these densities being, for all intents and purposes, totally black (Fig. 1.10).

This maximum density on a transmitted light image and the clarity of the base determine the maximum contrast available on the film, i.e. the blackest black and the whitest white. In other words, film can have a maximum density which is determined solely by the silver content and the value of the incident light.

With paper, however, different rules apply. Some incident light will *always* be reflected from the surface of the paper; it can never all be absorbed by the silver in the emulsion. Similarly to film, the maximum density is determined by the incident light, but this maximum density can be changed as it depends on the angle of the viewing light to the viewer and the surface of the paper, which can be glossy or matt (Fig. 1.11).

Because of these effects, film will always have a longer grey scale and a wider dynamic range than paper.

In the case outlined above, the discussion was about two similar processes for producing a hard copy of an image: however, there is another type of paper image which uses the *diffusion transfer process*. This should be considered separately.

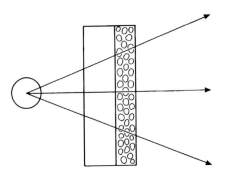

Fig. 1.10 The transmitted light passes straight through the film, generally only its intensity being reduced.

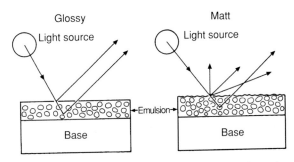

Fig. 1.11 With glossy paper there is reflection from the paper surface, then the light is reflected from the image. Matt paper suffers from multiple reflections from the coarse surface.

DIFFUSION TRANSFER PROCESS

The 'instant' picture is often used in ultrasound as a permanent record of the event. It is usually found as a paper image, in which case the same rules apply to this paper image as to conventional paper. It can also be found as a transmission image.

Pros and cons

When using diffusion transfer, some advantages and disadvantages of the system can be noted:

Advantages

1. No processing facilities required
2. 'Instant' viewing of finished image
3. High speed (can be approximately 3000 ISO)
4. Useful for museum or history of patient
5. No darkroom or darkroom equipment required.

Disadvantages

1. High cost per image
2. Low dynamic range (if paper)
3. Poor grey scale (if paper)
4. Can be messy to handle
5. Subject to ambient temperature levels.

However, none of the above should be taken to mean that diffusion transfer is unsatisfactory. Like many other processes in photography it has its place. It is up to individual users to decide which material suits a particular application.

WHY USE FILM?

Until very recently the ideal detector for X-rays was a photographic emulsion. The main advantages of film can be simply listed:

1. Film has a high emulsion sensitivity to short exposure times.
2. The natural spectral sensitivity of silver halide matches intensifying screen output.
3. Silver halide is capable of a high information density.
4. Silver halide produces a safe and permanent image (we still have images from the 1850s).

Perhaps the two main advantages can be put very simply:

1. *Film has extremely high spatial resolution.* It has very high resolving power, usually expressed in line pairs per millimetre (lp mm^{-1}). Film resolution can vary tremendously. With X-ray film, a typical figure would be 10 line pairs per millimetre.

2. *Film has extremely high temporal resolution.* It should not be forgotten that the extremely short radiographic exposures of today were only possible through the use of film. Film has the property of being able to freeze fast movement, providing enough energy is available.

It should be noted that to produce a *single* television frame requires 1/25 second. The image produced on the monitor must, of necessity, flicker. Many investigations have been done on the ergonomic design of a viewing station for prolonged reporting sessions, and much consideration has been given to this flicker in particular. Some manufacturers are considering using a monitor phosphor with an extended lag (i.e. after-glow) to try to reduce the flicker. Nonetheless, it is, at present, a problem.

Of course film – or more accurately silver halide – does have some disadvantages:

1. Only about 3–5% of the X-radiation is converted into a visible image
2. There is poor visualisation of low contrast subjects

3. Film requires 'offline' three-step wet processing
4. Erratic silver prices tend to destabilise film prices.

Perhaps the worst of these is the inability of film to cope with low contrast resolution, the ability to define very small differences in X-ray absorption.

Film versus electronics

One of the major attractions of electronic imaging, be it CT, ultrasound or any other form, is the fact that image processing, or manipulation, is extremely straightforward. Film does not allow this feature, at least not easily. In fact, the only real film image manipulation which may go on in the imaging department is subtraction.

Electronics do not have it all their own way. The main problems are interfacing (i.e. connecting one piece of apparatus to another) and ease of viewing. Film, on the other hand, can be posted, put into albums or viewed on a viewing box with consummate ease.

IMAGE COMPLEXITY

The first CT systems produced pictures on a square matrix of 80 × 80 pixels. Compared to today, this image was of very low resolution, using only 6400 pixels.

Matrices have increased in size over the years: first 320 × 320, then 512 × 512 and then 1024 × 1024. These figures give total numbers of pixels as 102 400, 262 144 and a staggering 1 048 576, respectively.

Initially magnetic tape, then disks were used to store the data, but it soon became apparent that the floppy disk could not handle the large volume of data produced.

In DSA, with a matrix of 1024 × 1024, one *10 second* study can generate 262 144 000 pixels at 25 frames per second. This very large number is further modified by the fact that every pixel is not just black or white, it is represented by varying shades of grey.

Considered at their most basic level, and ignoring any high level language which enables the user to communicate easily with them, computers use binary arithmetic. In other words, they simply count to two and start again.

In binary, 11111111 represents decimal 255; 00000001 represents decimal 1. If 2 is raised from the power 0 to 10, the following decimal numbers are obtained:

1; 2; 4; 8; 16; 32; 64; 128; 256; 512; 1024.

This helps to explain why these decimal numbers constantly recur in computerised imaging technology.

Taking a 512×512 matrix as an example, the matrix is made up of 512 vertical columns and 512 horizontal rows. At each pixel, the brightness level is converted to a binary number. Thus, if the pixel is able to demonstrate 256 brightness levels (2^8) then the pixel is said to be 8 bits deep. Zero will represent black and 255 will represent white.

It is, of course, possible to have a 7 bit deep pixel (128 brightness levels) or a 12 bit deep pixel (4096 brightness levels). Obviously the eye cannot see that number of grey levels, but it enables a very wide range of windowing levels to be used by the operator.

For example, if an image consists of 512×512 pixels, each 8 bits deep, then a total of 262 144 bytes are required.

The numbers required to record dynamic events are astronomical. Take for example a matrix 512×512, 8 bits deep, 25 frames a second and *a 1 second* event. This requires 6 553 600 bytes: so, for dynamic images on this type of matrix, almost 7 megabytes (Mbytes) a second are required.

PROCESSING

If the imaging camera does not contain an in-built processor, some consideration must be given to the processing of the final film. It should be remembered that an imaging film is single-sided emulsion film, and large quantities of this film going through the department's main processor could lead to gross over-replenishment. In some departments this decision is purely academic, as there may be only the one processor. In the purpose-built department there are a number of decisions to be made:

Automatic processing

The decision will revolve round the choice of low capacity, medium capacity or high capacity processors. Most imaging departments could cope with a low capacity processor, of the order of 30 cm/min running speed as the throughput of film is not as great as a 'normal' department. Nor is there the same demand to see the film quickly.

Darkroom availability should also be considered: ideally, the darkroom should be nearby, and the safelighting must be suitable for orthochromatic emulsions.

Daylight processing

Some manufacturers offer a cassette which is compatible with imaging cameras of other manufacturers. The same cassette can also be used in a daylight system, thus offering the additional advantages of daylight processing.

Quality assurance

Monitor photography film is much more susceptible to changes in processing quality than conventional screen film. The image quality will fluctuate quite markedly with chemical changes which would most probably be unnoticed on screen film. It is therefore very important to consider a quality assurance programme as routine. This would, of course, cover the camera as well as the processor.

Signal generators are now available which produce images suitable for evaluating image quality in cameras. These are extremely useful devices for the quality assurance of imagers.

One useful attribute of monitor photography is that testing of the camera and processor does not involve live patients. There is easy access to actual patients' images stored on disk, and these can be replayed time after time to assess image quality.

THE FINAL IMAGE

A common complaint is that the final hard copy does not look like the image on the diagnostic console. This can be due to many factors, not least the behaviour of the CRT itself.

The production of this final image is the result of a number of complex factors; the following is a short list of the most important:

Computer algorithms

These are instructions within the complex computer programs which translate the received information (the raw data) into a form usable by the diagnostic apparatus.

Monitor

The image display is a function of the video signal generated by the diagnostic apparatus. This, in turn, is determined by the characteristics of the monitor in use. Of course, some of these characteristics can be modified by the use of the brightness and contrast controls.

Film

This part of the process is determined by the characteristic curve of the film. However, this is inextricably linked with the CRT performance. For example, there are no truly linear relationships in this part of the imaging process. The relationship between log of intensity on the CRT display and the grid voltage means that low grid voltages give better contrast than higher grid voltages. The characteristic curve also is certainly not linear. In addition, it should be remembered that in most cases the film is imaging the reverse polarity of what is seen on the diagnostic monitor. The hard copy is essentially a compromise between all these factors.

There is also a disparity between the actual viewing sizes, for example between a large monitor and a relatively small format image.

The viewer's eye

The viewer's eye is perhaps the most complex part of the chain. The eye's response varies from viewer to viewer, as can easily be demonstrated by a Receiver Operating Characteristic test (see ROC, p. 184). In general, though, the human eye is much better at resolving density differences in the low rather than in the high density areas. Windowing can be used to exploit this effect.

COLOUR VERSUS BLACK AND WHITE

Coloured images are used to a limited extent in monitor photography. However, they are limited to specialised imaging, for example positron emission tomography (PET).

Part of the reason for the non-acceptance of colour as a universal image may lie in the fact that coloured imaging does not have a standard for colour values. Red may mean high density on one system and low density on another.

However, the use of colour could be very attractive: the human eye is capable of resolving only about 200 different grey levels, whereas it can discern about 2000 colour levels. These colour levels would be responded to in terms of colour hue and brightness levels.

Again, windowing can play a part in black and white imaging. Because most systems allow considerable windowing, the eye's ability to resolve only 200 grey levels is more than acceptable.

Colour also brings the problem of processing. Generally, the colour process is much more complex than black and white, and this is reflected in the price of the processors and film.

CONCLUSION

Monitor photography has become a mainstay of ultra-modern imaging. The development of this type of imaging is far from over, but monitor photography still uses a technology which is well over 150 years old and, because of the convenience of film, should continue to use it for some years to come. Film technology is developing continually and will continue to develop well into the foreseeable future. Electronic imaging, with its insatiable demand for hard copy, is more than established, yet it seems to have opened even more doors for film.

Chapter 2
The laser

INTRODUCTION

More and more images in imaging departments are being produced in an electronic form. They are initially viewed on a visual display unit. A variety of methods have been used to produce a hard copy of this information and at first the monitor was 'photographed' using either a Polaroid camera or a camera containing radiographic film. The growth of techniques such as ultrasound, CT scanning, nuclear magnetic resonance (NMR) and radionuclide imaging meant that each unit had to have its own equipment for image recording, thus increasing the expense. Laser imagers have combined the technology of the laser along with computer technology to enable the centralised production of hard copy images.

LIGHT AND THE LASER (Figs 2.1 and 2.2)

White light is made up of varying wavelengths, ranging from ultraviolet in the short wave, through visible light, to infrared in the long wavelengths. Because of the presence of all these wavelengths, white light has very short coherence lengths, due to the anti-phase components cancelling one another out.

The first laser was built in 1960, by Theodore Maiman, working at the Hughes Aircraft Electronic Research Laboratory. Maiman's laser was basically a photographer's electronic flashgun wound around a crystal of synthetic ruby (aluminium oxide mixed with a small amount of chromium). The synthetic ruby was in the form

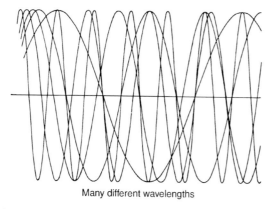

Many different wavelengths

Fig. 2.1 White light – a cacophony in vision.

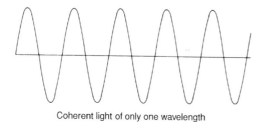

Coherent light of only one wavelength

Fig. 2.2 Laser light – coherent light of only one wavelength.

of a tube with a mirror at each end, one mirror being a partial reflector; the distance between the mirrors was precisely defined, as it was tuned to make the light produced bounce back and forth in a regular and reinforcing pattern to create standing waves of light in the rod (Fig. 2.3).

The operation of a laser

The mechanism of operation of a laser was not clearly understood until 1960. In basic terms it is simple:

- If a photon is fired at an atom, the atom can absorb the photon and thus be raised to an excited state. The only way that the atom can return to stability is by releasing this absorbed energy in the form of a photon of light (*spontaneous emission*).

- However, if a photon is fired at an already excited atom, the atom will release TWO light photons and then return to its stable state. This particular process is known as *stimulated emission*. In a laser, the atoms are stimulated by an external power source (Fig. 2.4).

- When a stage is reached whereby half the atoms are in an excited state, a situation known as *population inversion* occurs.

- If more photons are fired at this stage, *stimulated emission* takes place. Stimulated emission occurs at this point simply because it is more likely that the photons will strike an already excited atom rather than a stable atom (Fig. 2.5).

- If the events described occur in a tube, the tube can be 'tuned' to encourage the light produced to oscillate in a regular pattern, and to eventually break out as an extremely coherent, parallel beam of light which contains a considerable amount of energy.

LASER SOLUTIONS

When the laser first appeared it was referred to as a 'solution looking for a problem to solve'. Since then, the laser has indeed solved a great many problems. For example:

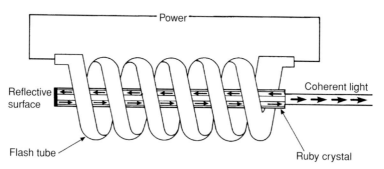

Power

Reflective surface

Coherent light

Flash tube

Ruby crystal

Fig. 2.3 Maiman's original synthetic ruby laser.

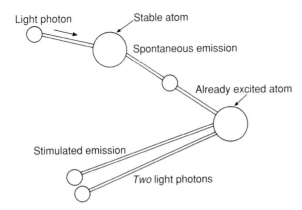

Fig. 2.4 Stimulated emission.

THE LASER IN MEDICINE

In medicine, lasers are used in a variety of applications, a few of which are listed below:

1. As surgical knives, as they cut and cauterise at the same time
2. To kill, very precisely, pre-cancerous cells in the neck of the cervix
3. To 'spot weld' the retina back into place
4. To treat veins in danger of haemorrhaging.

It is at the cellular level, however, that lasers have really come into their own. They can be focused so precisely (and yet carry such large amounts of power) that they can destroy a single cell, or even part of a cell. Lasers have been programmed by computers to recognise cancerous cells and destroy them.

Optical disks will certainly be used extensively in the digital imaging departments of the future. This development would have been impossible without the laser. In the compact disk, which contains digital musical information, a laser is used to read the digital pits created below the surface of the disk. At the introductory stage these disks were 'read' only (i.e. they could only be played

- The National Physical Laboratory has determined that the speed of light is exactly 186 282.397 miles per second, using a laser.

- Distance measurements accurate to one millionth of a centimetre can be made using a laser.

- When the Apollo astronauts left the moon, they left behind a mirror to reflect laser light. When laser light is bounced off this mirror, the distance of the earth to the moon can be determined to within an accuracy of 30 cm.

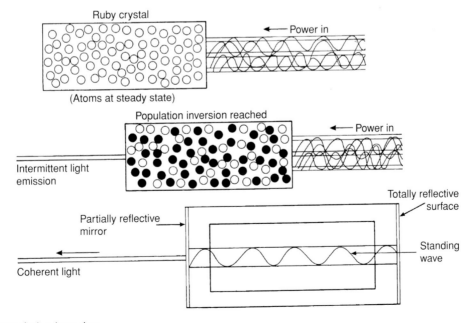

Fig. 2.5 Population inversion.

back). The information contained on the disks, however, was of very high quality. The large optical disk was then developed which was capable of playing back images. The modern version of these is capable of both reading and writing, that is the user can now record information on the disk. These disks are capable of very high storage capacity, typically 2.5 Gbytes.

The laser is used in these systems because it can be focused so accurately below the disk surface. This means that surface blemishes such as scratches will not be read by the laser. The laser also produces sufficient energy to deform the disk material so as to record the required information.

Pulsed or continuous

The laser that Maiman invented was a *pulsed laser*, and had a pulse of about three thousandths of a second.

The next major step forward was the *continuous wave gas laser* (Fig. 2.6), using helium and neon as the lasing material (see Laser imagers, p. 19). These lasers are extremely coherent and uniform, and can be switched off and on like a simple electric light.

LASER IMAGING

The laser imager is an optical/electronic/mechanical device which produces hard copy by exposing a film to laser light.

In the laser imager a helium-neon laser can be used, emitting red light. The principle of operation of the laser imager is entirely different from that of a video imager, even though the results obtained look remarkably similar.

Principles of operation

The laser imager contains a number of separate modules, all interlinked, which help in the production of the final image. They are:

1. The laser (usually helium-neon)
2. An interface
3. A large memory store
4. An acoustic-optical modulator
5. An optical system
6. A (mechanical) scanner
7. A (mechanical) film transport system.

Comparison between laser and video imaging

The memory store is required because image production on a laser imager is very different from that of a video imager. In a video imager, one image is captured on a CRT and photographed. In a laser imager *all* the digital image information required for one *film* must be put into the memory store, via the interface, before the image recording can start:

• The full information from the memory store is used to modulate the laser beam via an acoustic-optical modulator, in terms of brightness, grey levels, etc.

• A lens system is used to focus the laser beam onto a galvano scanner

• The scanner is used to move the laser beam from side to side across the imaging field.

In a video imager, writing the lines of information is achieved by the continuous deflection of the electron beam. In the laser imager the deflection of the beam in the horizontal plane is

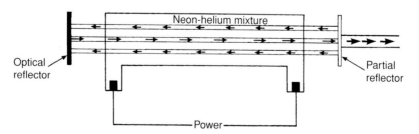

Fig. 2.6 Continuous wave gas laser.

achieved by a mirror. This leaves vertical movement, which has to be done by moving the film in relation to the deflected horizontal beam (Fig. 2.7).

LASER IMAGERS

Operator keypad

The operator keypad allows control of the parameters for imaging at the time of the examination. These can include:

- Film size
- Format, i.e. the number of images recorded on the film
- Image-store sequence
- Density
- Contrast
- Exposure
- Image polarity
- Clear or black border background
- Number of copies required
- Patient information
- Automatic hospital name, date recording
- Printing of the image.

It is also possible to delete an image prior to printing.

Input signal

The digital signal can be either transferred directly to the printer from the separate modalities or stored on computer disk and then taken to the laser imager. It is possible for the imagers to receive input signals at the same time as they are 'writing' an image, resulting in no processing delay.

Printing

Image storage

The image is stored in the RAM memory of the printer which has a basic memory capable of storing information to fill one 35×43 cm film from each modality at a time. When the memory is full, a film is automatically dispensed (by either gravity or rollers) and is positioned ready for scanning.

Scanning (Fig. 2.7)

Lasers produce coherent beams of parallel light and therefore the scanning optics can be much simpler than if white light is used which produces a divergent beam. Either a red, helium-neon laser which emits light of 632 nm or an infrared laser in the range of 750–850 nm can be used. The information from the memory store is used to modulate the laser beam in terms of brightness, grey scales, etc. and therefore the intensity of the beam will be determined by the digital value of the input signal.

Horizontal scanning. The beam is focused using an optical lens system onto a mirror system which moves the beam from side to side across the film, printing one line of information at a time. Each line is capable of containing between 3500 and 4100 pixels of information.

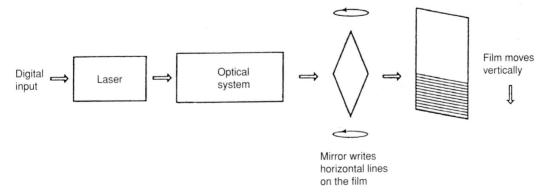

Fig. 2.7   Principles of a laser imager.

Vertical imaging. After each line has been printed, the film moves to allow the next line to be printed. Each film will have to move between 4250 and 5100 times before imaging has been completed.

The imaging process takes between 8 and 30 seconds.

Film characteristics

As the film is 'written on' by the laser, only a single-sided, fine grain, silver halide emulsion is required. This is mounted on either a blue tinted or a clear polyester base with an antihalation layer to prevent curl.

In order to obtain optimum results it is important that the correct film is purchased to match the type of laser used. Helium-neon lasers produce red light and therefore the film should have a sensitivity in the order of 633 nm, and special green safelight filters may be purchased if required for darkroom film handling. Infrared lasers require film with a sensitivity of between 780 and 850 nm and should be handled in total darkness. Fortunately, the film is packaged in such a way that it can be loaded into the laser printer in daylight conditions and from the printer it is automatically fed into the automatic processing unit.

Processing

When processing has been completed the film passes either directly to a conventional auto-matic processor or into a light-proof receiving magazine which is closed and taken to a separate automatic processor.

IMAGING PLATES

Imaging plates are now available for use in place of a conventional screen film combination.

Structure of the imaging plate
(Fig. 2.8)

1. *Protective layer*
    Thin, transparent film to protect the plate.

2. *Phosphor layer*
    Barium fluorohalide contained in a binder provides a photo-stimulable phosphor.

3. *Light reflection layer* (may be absent)
    Composed of light-reflecting particles in a binder.

4. *Conductive layer*
    Composed of conductive crystals in a binder. Its function is to reduce problems caused by electrostatic charges but in addition it absorbs light and therefore increases image sharpness.

5. *Support* (base)
    Has a similar structure and function to that of a conventional intensifying screen.

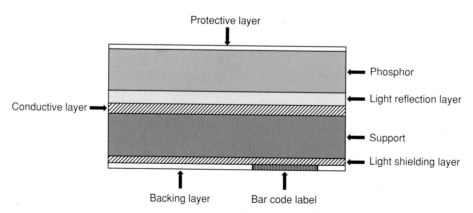

Fig. 2.8 Imaging plate.

6. *Light shielding layer*
   Composed of carbon particles in a binder and its function is to prevent light leaking from the backing area.

7. *Backing layer*
   A soft polymer layer to protect the plate during stacking of a number of imaging plates.

8. *Bar code label*
   Used to provide a serial number and to identify a particular imaging plate which can then be linked with patient identification details, etc. The code is printed on a piece of paper measuring 25 × 61 mm.

Cassettes

Imaging plates require special cassettes in order to protect them from damage. The cassettes look like conventional cassettes but with a window to allow reading of the imaging bar code.

Use of the imaging plate

Image erasure

The imaging plate is exposed to an erasing light to discharge any remaining energy from the previous exposure. The imaging plate is then ready for re-use.

Exposure

The imaging plate can be either loaded into the special cassette and employed in exactly the same way as a conventional screen-film combin-ation or used as part of a computed radiography system. When the plate is exposed to radiation, electrons are excited to higher energy levels in the barium fluorohalide phosphor crystals. The excited electrons are trapped in colour centres (F centres) which are halogen ion vacancies in the crystals.

Image reading (Fig. 2.9)

The cassette and imaging plate are then taken to the image recorder. If an imaging plate has been exposed but has not been read it should only be handled in conventional safelight conditions when the plate is being transferred to a magazine. If a computed radiography system is being used the plate will be automatically transported into the image recording unit.

A helium-neon laser scans the imaging plate and energy from the beam is absorbed by the plate. As a result the previously trapped electrons are released and recombine, thereby creating the phenomenon of photostimulated luminescence in the region of 400 nm.

PRINCIPLE OF PHOTOSTIMULATED LUMINESCENCE (Fig. 2.10)

The barium fluorohalide crystals have gaps (colour centres or F centres) in the higher energy levels. When the crystal is excited by radiation, electrons receive energy and move from the low energy, valency band to the colour centres in the high energy, conduction band. When the crystal

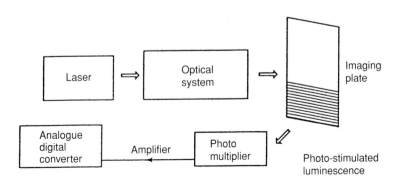

Fig. 2.9 Principles of image reading.

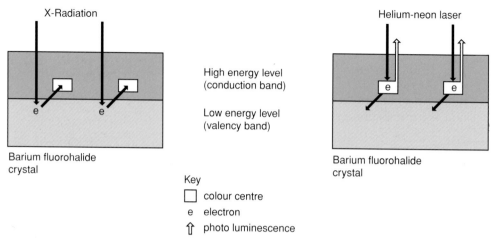

Fig. 2.10 Photostimulated luminescence.

is scanned by the helium-neon laser, energy is absorbed and then is released in the form of photoluminescence. This release of energy causes the electron to drop back to its former position in the valency band.

The luminescence is detected by the image detector (a photomultiplier) which converts it to time-series image signals. These are, in turn, converted into electrical signals, digitised and automatically transferred to a laser printer where they provide the input signal for the laser beam.

After printing, the process is similar to that of the laser imager; the film either passes directly and automatically to a conventional automatic processor or passes to a receiving magazine and is transported by hand.

DRY FILM PROCESSING

Technology is available which utilises direct laser printing to produce an image without the use of processing chemicals.

Film characteristics

The 12 × 24 cm film can be handled in daylight conditions and is either a blue or clear polyester-based film with a carbon coating. The carbon responds digitally to laser energy over a certain threshold value. Each pixel on the film contains in excess of 4000 sub-pixel elements called pels. The whole film has a scratch resistant 'overcoat'.

Imaging

The digital signal from the appropriate modality is fed into solid state laser diodes which then scan the film in a way similar to that of other laser printers. As the signal is digital, the pels are either exposed or not exposed and, as a result of their very small size and large numbers, shades of grey can be built up.

The film is ready for viewing in 90 seconds.

COMPARISON OF VIDEO AND LASER SYSTEMS (Fig. 2.11)

Resolution

In terms of resolution capability there is no comparison between a laser imager and a video imager; the laser imager is far better, with a resolution of 4000 × 5000 pixels, with 256 grey levels. However, this resolution is always on *one film*, not on *one image*, no matter how many images are on the film. Video imaging has a typical resolution of 1024 × 1024, but this resolution is the same on *every* image. It takes very little simple arithmetic to work out that if both systems have 12 images on a 35 × 43 cm film, the resolution of both systems is virtually identical.

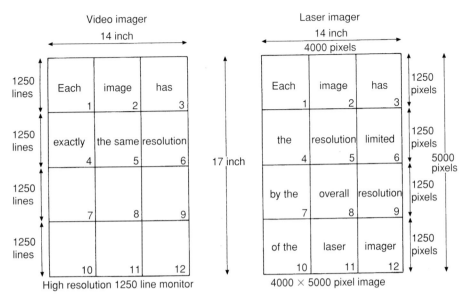

Fig. 2.11 Comparison of laser and video imagers.

Transfer of data

In data transmission terms: a typical transfer time of a video imager would be 40 ms. In a laser imager, which relies on digital transmission, a transfer time would be of the order of 8–30 seconds.

Exposure control

Exposure controls on a video imager are brightness, contrast and time of exposure. With a laser imager the image can be manipulated and the parameters changed prior to printing.

Film sizing

At present all major manufacturers seem to be making film for laser imagers. The film sizes available are:

35×43 cm
35×35 cm
24×24 cm
11×14 in
10×12 in
8×10 in

Some manufacturers have a laser imager using infrared film, whereas other manufacturers have opted for a conventional film technology.

Disadvantages/advantages

Video imagers can be affected by strong magnetic fields. In MRI, for example, this can cause problems unless due consideration is given to the siting and shielding of the imager in relation to the MRI apparatus. Also, the phosphor coating on the CRT is sometimes not uniform, giving rise to areas of low or high intensity on the image.

The laser imager is very susceptible to dust and vibration, particularly as the laser beam transfer is via a mirror. Additionally the vertical movement of the film by mechanical means must remain absolutely in register throughout the whole of the exposure. Any interruption of this travel, caused by vibration or mechanical movement, will produce gross artefacts on the image.

However, as the optics for laser imagers are fairly simple there tends to be less image distortion.

Which is best?

The laser imager produces superior images when used as a large format single image. However, this image must be produced from a high resolution matrix of 2048×2048 or greater. To use a matrix resolution of 512×512 on a unit capable of 4000×5000 resolution in large format would be patently absurd. However, digital radiography is rapidly requiring just this sort of high resolution area, coupled with the benefit of large grey scale levels in the order of 256 shades of grey.

Video imaging has a large part to play in general imaging, where its resolution capabilities fit in well with the demands of present day systems. The consistent resolution of the image, no matter how many images are on one film, weighs heavily on the side of video imaging. The short wait times for the image to be produced are also greatly in its favour.

For very high resolution digital radiography composed of a large single format image, the laser imager is preferred. However, laser imagers are expensive in comparison with video imagers.

CONCLUSION

There is no doubt that the advent of the laser has revolutionised the work of imaging departments. Laser printers have enabled the rapid manipulation, transfer and processing of images. The advent of imaging plates has meant that the concept of a filmless department has become a reality. The aim of this chapter has been to give a basic grounding of the principles on which the reader can then build and, it is hoped, understand the advances which may well appear in the future.

Chapter 3
Computing

CHAPTER CONTENTS

INTRODUCTION

In recent years computers have been ubiquitous, appearing on items as diverse as CT scanners and ultrasound units and computers that cope with the day-to-day running of patient records in reception. With so many developments in information exchange, the computer has become an important item in the imaging department, both in the process of imaging itself and in the collation of statistical information.

In order to operate, computers have to be programmed in a language they understand. A brief description of computer programming language is included in this chapter, and the second half of the chapter relates to a management system for an imaging department, an overview of networking and three-dimensional imaging. While a chapter such as this can never hope to be comprehensive, it will serve as an introduction to the technology.

THE SILICON CHIP

Silicon has been the basis of the chip for many years. The relative price of silicon is the same now as it was almost thirty years ago, but many more thousands of chips can now be put onto a 4 in disk.

However, the development of satellite television has placed extreme demands on silicon; for this purpose, gallium arsenide is replacing silicon. Since gallium arsenide is much faster than silicon, it offers a big advantage in computing.

Printing the chip

Microchips are basically printed, using a form of photography, through a photo-resist and directly onto the chip material. The final resolution of this process is important, as the final result is basically produced by reducing a large negative to a microscopically small size. The printing of the circuitry originally used ultraviolet (UV) light as the printing light: this gives a typical final resolution of 1/1000 of a millimetre. If, instead of UV, beams of electrons are used to print, the resolution is doubled.

However, both of these methods suffer from scatter within the photographic medium, and experimentation has suggested that *heavy ion* imaging would produce finer detail and permit 'ballistic transfer' of electrons, as the chip would be very small indeed. ('Ballistic transfer' means that the distances within the chip are so small that the electrons travel like bullets to their destination, without even atoms intervening in their path.)

In one research laboratory, it has been proved that 100 000 000 single transistors can be printed per square *millimetre* – or, to put it another way, 20 bibles could be printed on a pinhead!

The implication of this development was enormous as it resulted in the production of much smaller microchips. This, in turn, has resulted in the manufacture of much faster and smaller computers.

The computer has evolved very rapidly indeed, perhaps more rapidly than any other comparative technology, and the process will no doubt continue.

COMPUTER LANGUAGES

Machine code

When computers first arrived on the scene, the inputs and outputs were on paper tape and involved laborious calculations to turn the instructions into binary arithmetic (machine code), the *only* language that a computer understands.

It became obvious to everyone that unless there were a great many mathematical geniuses around, computers would stay in universities and laboratories and would remain inaccessible to the general public. High level languages for computers were therefore developed.

High level languages

A high level language can be defined as a language in which each instruction or statement (in almost plain English) corresponds to several machine code instructions.

BASIC has become the most common of the high level languages. BASIC was initiated by the US company Microsoft. Unfortunately, the language of BASIC has many dialects and this generally means that a program written in one dialect of BASIC will not run on another.

BASIC reserved words

To enable any computer to RUN it must have some form of language for it to be able to LOAD a program. You may wish to SAVE the program onto disk or tape. It may also be necessary in the program for the computer to READ a set of DATA and, from time to time, GOTO various sections of the program to be able to LIST certain variables which have been turned into STRING$.

You may also have to WAIT WHILE the computer WENDS its way through very long CHAINs of numbers before it can RESTORE itself and RETURN to the program and allow you to INPUT more information before it will PRINT out the name you wanted to DELETE. Eventually the program will STOP, END and finally CLOSE.

Admittedly, the above two paragraphs are contrived, but all of the words in capitals are 'reserved words' in BASIC; they give a computer specific instructions as to what to do. BASIC is an almost universal language among home computers, mainly due to the simplicity of programming in the BASIC language.

Exactly the same constraints are put on all high level languages. It is impossible to use these words within a program without the computer translating them into a piece of specific instruction.

Unfortunately, BASIC is unsuitable for large scale programming as, in computer terms, it is very slow. This is due to the fact that all the instructions given in BASIC have to be translated into machine code by the computer.

Portability

Simple programs can be written on most of the popular computers in a fairly standard BASIC, using the same reserved words. However, these programs, even though they use the same notations, are not *portable* – i.e. the recorded program will *not* run on a different machine.

However, once the realm of BASIC is left behind, this situation changes quite considerably. For example, CP/M is a fairly standard 'business' computer language. Any computer capable of running CP/M is capable of running any program written in that language.

Syntax

The BASIC language, which most people have some knowledge of, provides an excellent example of the use of syntax.

Like any foreign language, the BASIC language has its own syntax which differs from that of English. In some dialects of BASIC, for example, the word GOTO can only be entered as GOTO, not GO TO. The computer may reject one or other version as incorrect. Similarly, a comma (,) or a colon (:) or double quotes (") all have their own parts to play. Without the correct insertion of specific punctuation and words, the program will simply refuse to run.

DICOM

Computer systems have developed independently and therefore are unable fully to communicate with each other. DICOM stands for Digital Imaging and Communications in Medicine and is an initiative sponsored by the Radiological Society of North America and the Health and Management Systems Society. The aim of the initiative is to integrate information and management systems so that clinical information can be communicated among all specialities and providers. Ultimately this will mean that any doctor will have access to a wide range of tests and images which can be seen on a computer during consultation with any patient. The primary concern with this integration is one of patient confidentiality, but it can be argued that this system will reduce the number of times that patient information is manually handled and the security of the information can be assured by the use of passwords and security systems. In addition, it is possible to build in a system of monitoring access to each piece of information and to produce an audit trail of when the information has been accessed, for how long and by using which password. Major manufacturers are signed up to this initiative and all new systems should be checked to ensure that they are using DICOM.

BINARY

The words 'bit' and 'byte' are a description of how computers store and manipulate numbers.

We are taught to manipulate numbers in base 10. Computers, being simple devices, can only handle a 0 or a 1. Binary arithmetic is thus ideal for computers, because it counts to the base 2 instead of 10; '01 plus 10' = 3. This enables very large numbers to be represented by a series of ones and zeros, e.g. 01110111 is the binary equivalent of 119.

The smallest piece of information that a computer can handle is called a 'bit', derived from BInary digiT. This 'bit' is represented by a simple electrical signal. An electrical signal can either be ON or OFF; the 'bit' can therefore be represented by an 'ON' or 'OFF' signal.

Consider a row of two simple switches, each of which can be ON or OFF. There can only be the following four possible states:

OFF OFF or 0 0 (decimal 0)

[or]

OFF ON or 0 1 (decimal 1)

[or]

ON OFF or 1 0 (decimal 2)

[or]

ON ON or 1 1 (decimal 3)

Four different states is a very small range of numbers. In binary this could only represent the (decimal) numbers from 0 to 3.

If eight switches are used, the higher decimal numbers could be displayed. If all the switches were on they would represent the following decimal total:

ON	ON	ON	ON	ON	ON	ON	ON
128	64	32	16	8	4	2	1

The values add up to 255.

Now consider the same row of switches, some switches ON and some OFF, in the positions illustrated:

ON OFF ON OFF ON OFF OFF ON

Now substitute binary numbers in place of the switching states, and the row becomes:

ON	OFF	ON	OFF	ON	OFF	OFF	ON
1	0	1	0	1	0	0	1

Translating the binary numbers into their decimal equivalents, the values are:

ON	OFF	ON	OFF	ON	OFF	OFF	ON
1	0	1	0	1	0	0	1
128	0	32	0	8	0	0	1

Thus the decimal equivalent of:

1	0	1	0	1	0	0	1

is the sum of the 'ON' switches, or the binary 1s, i.e. 128 + 32 + 8 + 1, or 169.

In other words, in binary, these eight switches can now show all the numbers between 0 and 255 inclusive, or 256 separate states.

When eight of these 'bits' are grouped together they are known as a 'byte' and each byte is a unique combination of zeros and ones.

When a computer stores this byte, it effectively means that a number between 0 and 255 is stored, in binary form, in a specific location within the computer's memory.

In certain computers, for example, if sophisticated graphics are used, they are created using binary code and then used as data by the computer.

However, the main use for the numbers 0 to 255 is in the ASCII code to designate numbers, characters and symbols used on the computer keyboard.

HEXADECIMAL

Another type of numbering is the hexadecimal system, which uses base 16. Hexadecimal is unusual in that it uses numbers and letters in the notation. Decimal numbers from 0 to 20 are listed in Table 3.1 to illustrate the big differences between decimal, hexadecimal and binary systems.

DEPARTMENTAL MANAGEMENT WITH A COMPUTER

A senior consultant radiologist listed the requirements for a computer system for an imaging department. The main points are listed below:

Reduce repetitive tasks

With a computer installed in the department, routine and repetitive form-filling should become a thing of the past. For example, once a patient's name has been entered, it should not be necessary to have to re-enter it.

Reduce paper handling and filing

While the paperless department will not be with us for many years to come, a considerable reduction can be expected in jobs such as filing or storage of (paper) details of patients, etc.

Table 3.1 Comparison of decimal, hexadecimal and binary number systems 0–20		
Decimal	Hexadecimal	Binary
0	0	0
1	1	1
2	2	10
3	3	11
4	4	100
5	5	101
6	6	110
7	7	111
8	8	1000
9	9	1001
10	A	1010
11	B	1011
12	C	1100
13	D	1101
14	E	1110
15	F	1111
16	10	10000
17	11	10001
18	12	10010
19	13	10011
20	14	10100

Improve interdepartmental communication

Ready access is assured, with the proviso of password protection, to all the necessary details which enable departments to run smoothly.

Improve efficiency

A computer system can considerably increase the overall efficiency of departments.

Improve confidentiality and security

Files, reports and patient details can be very secure. To try and retrieve details without a password, or knowledge of the system, would be made very difficult.

Automate data collection

With a computer system, retrieval of all data can be accomplished 'at the touch of a button'. With the need to collect and handle a large volume of data the use of a computer is essential. Clinical budgeting can be very successfully helped by a computer.

A management computer installed in an imaging department should also be able to supply the following ancillary functions:

Research

Patient details and their films could be retrieved easily, and, using some simple identifying procedure, information could be obtained which would prove invaluable for research purposes or for the compilation of teaching cases.

Spreadsheet

The increasing demands of clinical budgeting could be well-supported using a spreadsheet, an electronic accounting ledger which can project 'what if' calculations with ease.

Word processing

Most people who have used a word processor would never go back to a conventional typewriter. On a word processor, routine letters, requests, etc., can be stored for immediate printout.

The use of a computer for departmental management can bring many benefits. It is worth looking in detail at some of the aspects which can bring considerable improvements to a modern imaging department.

Patient enquiries

In a major London teaching hospital, a survey was conducted into the number of patient enquiries passing through the department per day. These were enquiries such as:

'Have you the report on ....?'
'Has he arrived ....?'
'Can we have the films for ...?'
'Have you got the films for ...?'
'Can we make an appointment for ...?'

The enquiries were broken down as follows:

Phone   90
Appointments   65

Arrival	300
Report request	35
Film request	450
Total	940

At the end of the day, 940 patient enquiries had been made. The average response time to answer these queries was 55 seconds.

Nine hundred and forty queries at an average of 55 seconds adds up to 14.36 person hours per day!

Using a computer, which should have an average response time of significantly less than 5 seconds, the 940 queries can be tackled in about 2 person hours per day. This represents a saving of more than 12 person hours per day.

A computerised film store

How can a computer help in film store management – a major problem in many departments?

The use of a computer enables sequential filing to take place. This means that at the end of a day's session, the films are filed sequentially and placed in the file in that particular day's slot. Eventually a 'hot' area is created at the end of the file, where the most frequent attenders will be found, and a 'cold' area where all of the 'dead' films will eventually arrive.

Apart from being extremely simple and quick to use, sequential filing offers a very high degree of security, as the films are filed under days rather than under a hospital or computer number. No longer can films be removed furtively. Unless the location is known, the films are virtually impossible to find. Sequential filing, which is used by many large companies with vast indexes, is only really manageable with a fast computer which is able to store and retrieve locations quickly.

Table 3.2 compares a manual and a computer-controlled film store system.

Table 3.2 Comparison of manual and computer-controlled film storage systems

	Manual system	Computer-controlled system
Patient attends	*Search* for old films: If found, fill in tracer and exchange	Computer confirms presence or absence of films
	If not found, make a new packet	If they exist, current film location shown
Examination completed	*Search* for tracer and exchange	Place film at end of file
Patient attends clinic	*Search* for packet:	Computer indicates films location
	If found, fill in tracer and exchange	*Search* file for films
Films returned to store	*Search* for tracer and exchange	Place films at *end* of file
Patient never seen again	*Search* for 'dead' films and remove	'Dead' films at *beginning* of files

Summary		
	Manual system	Computer-controlled system
	5+ *Searches* for film packet	All films in sequence of acquisition
	Misfiles easy = *total loss*	A computer can record date (even bin number)
	Search essential to determine presence/absence of films	'Hot' store for films most likely to be pulled
	Requires tracer cards	Refiles *always* at end of file
	No immediately available record of outstanding films and their destinations and durations	A computer can give file date, or location and date if film is out of the files

NETWORKING

Networking is a method of linking imaging systems throughout an organisation to allow the rapid transfer of information between computers. It is possible to purchase and install a variety of interlinked units to meet individual needs. The first 'filmless' hospital was opened in the UK in July 1992 at the Conquest Hospital in Hastings; this was only made possible by the use of networking.

Economics of the 'filmless department'

When a new department is being commissioned, a decision has to be made whether or not to go down the 'filmless route'; perhaps, therefore, it is worth looking at some of the considerations for a 'filmless department':

Considerations

- The system selected should be easy to use
- The image archive must be secure and there must be no loss of image quality during storage
- Archived images can be compressed for ease of storage but there should be no loss of data on compression
- The system selected should not tie the department to the use of a specific equipment manufacturer
- Old hard copy images need to be converted to the new system.

Advantages

- Rapid image access
- Rapid film filing and retrieval
- Rapid transportation within the hospital (and, if the technology is in place, between other hospitals and e.g. GP fund holders)
- If a dry film system is used for hard copies, no chemicals, silver recovery or waste disposal problems
- A potential 40% saving on the film and chemical bill

- Image manipulation possible and therefore a potential for reducing patient dosage
- Instant availability of images for reporting is possible
- Archived images can be compressed for ease of storage
- Reduction of storage space required
- Ability to view the same image at two different sites simultaneously, leading to quicker reporting on films created in satellite units
- The manual transportation of films is not required.

Disadvantages

- Hard copies will still be required, especially if a patient is transferred to a 'conventional' department
- Initial installation cost is high
- Needs to be linked throughout the health community to be totally effective
- Requires full integration with the radiology and hospital information systems to gain maximum benefit.

PICTURE ARCHIVING AND COMMUNICATION SYSTEMS (PACS)

PACS is a method of storing images in a digital format. Once stored they can be sent to different parts of the hospital and to the wider medical community. Many manufacturers produce systems to enable the transfer of information and the systems they produce contain some or all of the following:

Image identification

- Either a bar code reader or a touch screen for patient identification
- Either a bar code reader or a touch screen for cassette identification.

This can be either downloaded from the central hospital computer or appropriate imaging modality, keyed in using the computer keyboard, or directly read from a bar code.

Reporting consoles

Reporting consoles allow instant access to diagnostic images, allowing the decision to be taken immediately as to whether or not additional projections will be required before the patient leaves the department. In addition, current and archived images and previous reports can be displayed alongside each other to give a full clinical picture of the patient's condition prior to reporting.

It is possible to change the image presentation on the monitor with regard to the following:

- *Viewing* several images together

- *Viewing* an animated sequence of images

- *Tonal conversion*: the selection of the appropriate contrast and density for the anatomical region under investigation

- *Spatial frequency modification*: this allows the selective manipulation of an image to eliminate 'blurring' or contrast disparity

- *Edge enhancement*: as the name suggests, this more clearly defines the outline of various bones or organs

- *Magnification*: this allows different parts of the image to be magnified, although some systems do not allow the magnified image to be recorded on film

- *Measurement, rotation and image reversal*: these are all possible and in some instances the operator is able to manipulate the image to produce three-dimensional images providing the appropriate software and images are present

- *Sound reporting*: this is the means of dictating and then saving an oral report by using a telephone headset. The recording can then be digitised and stored with the appropriate image. The recording can then be archived, transmitted or replayed at a later date.

Remote consoles

These can be:

- Viewing stations to retrieve images from the intranet for internal staff
- Viewing stations to retrieve information from the internet for external staff.

The consoles can be sited throughout the hospital: in intensive care units, theatres, accident and emergency departments, teaching units, etc. The images can be displayed alongside the reports and additional information (e.g. exposure factors) can also be displayed. The use of these consoles can save time as the manual retrieving, transporting and copying of films is no longer required.

Central storage

A web server with a database to store the image

- With automatic deletion after the patient leaves hospital.

A web browser

- For the selection of information by patient name
- For the selection of images of a specific patient.

Storage in a DICOM format

- Allows universal connections to imagers, workstations and external users

- Using either RAID (redundant array of independent discs) or CD-R or digital linear tape (DLT).

Computerised archiving

It is possible to create a database for each patient entering the hospital. This is used to record patient information, current history, referral letters (which may be received directly from the GP via an electronic mailing system), test results, reports and an accounting system (to enable rapid and accurate invoicing). In addition it is possible automatically to create statistical information for stock control and for ordering new equipment. Patient information can remain in the system until the patient is discharged from the hospital and can then be automatically stored in the central archive. As it is possible to store in the order of 2500 diagnostic images on a $5\frac{1}{4}$ in optical disk, or up to 15 000 images on a 12 in optical disk, there can be a large saving in storage space.

Information retrieval can be based on patient surname/forenames, date of birth, imaging number, condition, date of imaging production or audit value.

Hard copy images

By networking the system to a laser printer it is possible to select and then produce hard copies of images and reports for storage in the patient's notes in the conventional way.

Modem links

A modem is the term used for an interface which links units via the telephone system. It can be used to send images to other hospitals, either in this country or abroad. For example, if a patient was to have an accident on the continent and then return to the UK, the images and reports could be transmitted directly to the receiving hospital. Or if a patient had a condition diagnosed in one hospital and needed to be transfered to a specialist unit, again the images could be sent directly.

Some installations allow direct connection to a service engineer to allow the engineer to do quality control checks or to trace and, in some instances, rectify software faults. If faults occur in the hardware, remote fault diagnosis may also be possible, enabling the engineer to order the appropriate components and coordinate the arrival of the parts and the engineer to minimise departmental down-time.

Image security

- Via passwords and defined user groups
- External sources receive encoded data.

Automatic updating

- Enables the system to automatically access new innovations and technology.

THREE-DIMENSIONAL IMAGING

With the advent of workstation systems with their associated increase in power and memory, at an affordable price, software packages have been developed which enable the production of three-dimensional images which can be displayed, manipulated and allow measurements to take place. In a networked system it is now possible to manipulate images at stand-alone workstations by, if necessary, downloading power to prevent system overload. Software can be used to manipulate images from ultrasound, CT, MRI, etc. to aid with, for example, radiotherapy planning, joint replacement surgery, cosmetic surgery and tracing major vessels prior to operations. It is also possible to combine images from several modalities and, for example, enhance the image or change its orientation.

Application

Volume measurements

These can be in the form of quantitative analysis of a defined area, for example a tumour, and statistical analysis could be performed and the results presented graphically if required.

Curved sections

By selecting a standard plane through the body which could be transverse, coronal or sagittal, a curved line could be drawn. This could, for example, follow a blood vessel, and therefore its relationship with the associated structures could be identified.

Volume rendered images

By adjusting the threshold values of an image, either the soft tissue, bone structure or internal organs can be displayed from the same original image.

Image enhancement

This could be used to manipulate an under-exposed image to make it diagnostically accept-able. There is therefore the potential for reducing the initial patient dosage and, by reading, and then manipulating the image from an imaging plate, producing a diagnostic image.

IMAGE ANALYSIS

It is now possible to undertake computer analy-sis of X-ray film images. Some example of how this technology is being utilised are described below:

Pronosco X-posure System™

This is a method of assessing bone mineral dens-ity:

- The hand, wrist and forearm are radiographed

- The radiograph is digitised using a scanner system

- The radius, ulna and three middle metacarpal bones are automatically analysed for porosity and striation

- A printout of the bone mineral density estim-ate is produced.

ImageChecker™

To aid with the screening of routine mammo-grams:

- The mammograms are taken

- The films are placed in an image checker proces-sor which contains a bar code reader, a laser film digitizer and a computer to process the images

- The image is digitised

- The image is automatically analysed to show regions of interest

- Clusters of white areas are marked

- Dense areas with radiating lines are marked

- The original films are reported on in the nor-mal way

- The display unit is then activated and the marked images are displayed

- The radiologist then reviews the original films in the light of the additional information.

The above examples merely illustrate some of the benefits that computers can bring into an imaging department. The systems currently on offer vary tremendously in size and therefore capacity, and in the functions they are able to undertake. Some systems are capable of using and generating bar codes, which enable much quicker entry into the computer and reduce the keyboard skills required by the users (they also considerably reduce the opportunities for error).

Larger systems are capable of storing vast amounts of data; indeed, some are capable of storing patient reports and film details for up to a million patients.

IMAGE STORAGE

There are a variety of storage methods in use, and it is worth considering the figures for each in turn.

Magnetic disk

A typical 8 in (double density, double sided) disk can hold about 1.2 Mbytes, i.e. four 512×512 images.

Magnetic tape

A 2400 ft tape can hold 180 Mbytes. That repre-sents storage for about:

- Six hundred and eighty-five 512×512 images
- 2.3 10-second studies
- Eleven 17×14 in film images.

Additionally, it can take nearly 4 minutes to find a specific image on the tape.

Optical disk storage

It is expected that a double-sided optical disk can hold about 2.5 gigabytes (Gbytes): that is, 2.5 bil-lion bytes.

For straightforward data storage, i.e. text, that is a large amount of storage capacity. To try and put this figure into perspective, a capacity of 600 Mbytes, or only 0.6 Gbytes, would be capable of storing all details, reports, film locations, appointments, X-ray room details, registrations, etc., for about a million patients. That represents the storage of all patient data (in an average hospital) for about 10 years. However, the storage of images is a different matter.

Even 2.5 Gbytes is only capable of handling about 170 35×43 cm (17×14 in) chest films. Data compression can be considered at this stage, although it can be difficult to implement. Typical data compression may be able to reduce storage requirements by as much as 50%. Even so, large numbers of optical disks would be required to store all the images archived in a busy general hospital, bearing in mind that statistics say that about 30% of work in a general department is chests.

The main factor in favour of the optical disk is the fact that *once it is filled*, any image can be found in about a quarter of a second.

The transmission of these large amounts of data to a remote viewing area should also be considered. The transmission of 2.5 Gbytes at even 1 Mbyte a second takes a significant amount of time if the transfer is by hard wire. If optical transmission, by optical fibre, is considered, this transfer time will reduce considerably. However, the installation of optical fibres, even if available, is an expensive exercise.

A 15 Mbyte PROM

This is a solid state, large-scale integrated detection-display device, sensitive to a wide range of the general electromagnetic spectrum. The device is flexible and allows excellent archiveability. The device can be viewed without any electronic display system or computer. It is totally portable and is easily transmitted. The device has a capacity of 15 Mbytes, and a density of 10^9 bits/cm^2. The device is extremely inexpensive.

Reading the above description, the device appears totally revolutionary; however, this inexpensive PROM (programmable *read only memory*) is a 35×43 cm (17×14 in) film. (This description assumes that the film is digitised to 0.1 mm pixels.)

If X-ray images are recorded onto a 35×43 cm (17×14 in) film, 15 Mbytes are immediately available to a radiologist, in a form which the eye and brain can easily process and interpret. If these images are microfilmed and 20 of them are recorded onto a 12×43 cm (5×17 in) film, we have the equivalent of 300 Mbytes (0.3 Gbytes).

It seems, from today's viewpoint, that film still has a future in the imaging department. It is also inevitable that digital equipment will appear in great numbers, although the full implementation of digital equipment will remain costly.

CONCLUSION

It seems inevitable that computers, in many forms and guises, will occupy a major place within imaging departments of the future, not simply in management but also in imaging technology. It is very difficult to determine where their future influence may lie: they have already made an impact on imaging in general, and other uses for them may well arise.

REFERENCE

Meire H B 1986 Private communication.

Chapter 4
Film materials

INTRODUCTION

The main aim of this chapter is to discuss the structures of film, basic film types and the manufacturing process; however, emulsion technology is a rapidly developing area and by the time this book reaches print other developments and advances may well have been made.

ELECTROMAGNETIC SPECTRUM

For a full description of the electromagnetic spectrum the reader is referred to any good physics text book. The following is intended to act as revision of the basic principles and only contains sufficient information to enable understanding of the rest of the text.

By definition, the electromagnetic spectrum is 'the range of frequencies over which electromagnetic radiation can be propagated' (*Penguin Dictionary of Physics* 1979). It ranges from the low frequencies that are associated with radio waves, to cosmic rays that have higher and higher frequencies. Figure 4.1 shows the electromagnetic spectrum with its common divisions and subdivisions. In general we are concerned with the frequencies between 10^{12} Hz and 10^{22} Hz, but in many cases, as in the chapter on screens (Ch. 5) for example, discussion will take place in terms of wavelengths in nanometers (nanometer = 10^{-9} m).

Electromagnetic radiation

Electromagnetic radiation is radiation consisting of waves of energy that are caused by the acceleration of charged particles. They consist of electric and magnetic fields that are propagated at right angles to each other and to the direction of propagation. The vibration causing the waves is sinusoidal and, unlike sound waves for example, electromagnetic waves require no supporting medium for their transfer. In free space (i.e. a vacuum) they travel at a uniform velocity of 2.997925×10^{8} m/s. The nature of electromagnetic radiation depends on its frequency (f) and its velocity (c), the relationship being that

$$c = f \lambda$$

where λ is the wavelength (Fig. 4.2).

It would probably all be quite simple if it ended here, but unfortunately when observed phenomena are being explained it is necessary to use either the *wave* concept of electromagnetic radiation or the *particle* concept of electromagnetic radiation (i.e. quantum theory). This is due to the fact that some phenomena, such as reflection, refraction and interference, can be explained using wave theory while other phenomena, such as the photoelectric effect and absorption, require an explanation in terms of particles.

The basis of the wave theory has already been discussed. It is based on the premise that electromagnetic radiation is propagated in the form of sinusoidal waves consisting of an electric field with its associated magnetic field at right angles to it and also at right angles to the direction of propagation. Figure 4.2 illustrates this and the 'cardinal' points of the sinusoidal wave, such as amplitude, wavelength, etc. Since all electromagnetic radiations have the same velocity, it follows that the frequency is inversely proportional to the wavelength. Wavelength may vary from miles, as in certain radio waves, to billionths of a metre, as in X-rays.

Particle theory

The particle theory of electromagnetic radiation is the basis of the concept of quantum physics. It

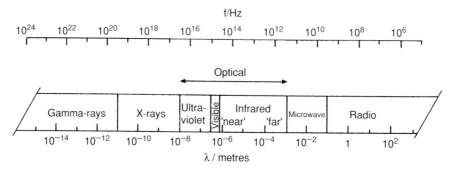

Fig. 4.1   The electromagnetic spectrum.

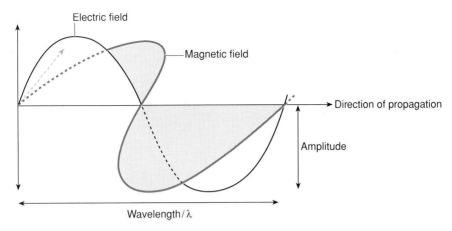

Fig. 4.2 Electromagnetic radiation.

applies particularly to 'waves' of short wave-length and high velocity which can be consid-ered as consisting of a stream of particles, or quanta, each having a discrete amount of energy (alternatively, these quanta may be known as photons). The amount of energy (E) carried in this discrete parcel is described by the formula:

$$E = hf$$

where:

E = energy
h = Planck's constant
f = frequency of the radiation

Planck's constant has been determined by experiment to be 4.13×10^{-18} keV.s or 6.626196×10^{-34} Js.

As the velocity of the particle in this case is constant, if the frequency of the radiation is doubled the energy of the photon is also doubled.

Throughout the text the principle used to describe physical processes will be the particle theory. On some occasions, however, use will be made of the wave theory, but this will be largely when dealing with optics.

VISIBLE SPECTRUM

Figure 4.1 shows that the visible spectrum occu-pies only a minute portion of the whole range of the electromagnetic spectrum. It is called the vis-ible spectrum because it is the range of wave-lengths within which the unaided human eye perceives wavelength changes as an alteration in colour. The extent of this spectrum is approxi-mately 400–700 nanometers (nm) and is a gradual change in colour from violet (400 nm) through to red (700 nm approximately), encompassing all the colours of the rainbow. Traditionally it is con-veniently divided into seven colours, as illus-trated in Figure 4.3, but it must be remembered that no sharp delineation occurs between each of the stated colours. There is some sensitivity of the eye to wavelengths outside the 'normal' range, down to about 380 nm (just ultraviolet) at the shorter wavelengths and up to about 780 nm (just infrared) at the longer wavelengths.

The value of the longest wavelengths to which the eye is sensitive is dependent on the 'bright-ness' of the 'object'. It can be extended up to 900 nm if a very high-power light source is used, but this is an extreme example.

Conventional photography is mainly con-cerned with a film's response to the visible spec-trum and conveniently divides the spectrum up into three areas or bands:

1. 400–500 nm, blue violet
2. 500–600 nm, green
3. 600–700 nm, red.

This is only an approximate division, but for many practical purposes it holds true.

In radiography our concern is not only with the visible spectrum but also with the effects on

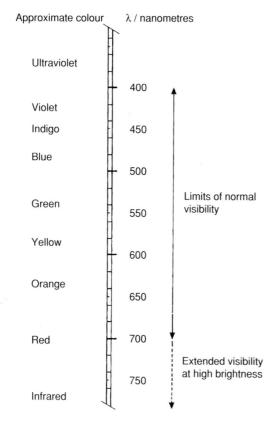

Fig. 4.3 The visible spectrum.

the film of ultraviolet, X- and gamma rays. This is frequently further complicated by the fact that most images are built up by a combination of differing effects depending on the different parts of the electromagnetic spectrum to which the film is exposed, for example a conventional film and X-ray intensifying screen produce an image that is made up partly of the effects of blue/green light exposing the film and partly of effects of direct X-ray exposure.

Each of these effects, and any effects they may have on each other, must be considered if an accurate assessment of how the image has been formed is to be made.

STRUCTURE OF THE FILM EMULSION

The film emulsion is the basic 'sensitive material' used to record the image. It is a suspension of a suitable light-sensitive salt (i.e. the silver halides) within a gelatine binder. Conventionally this suspension is coated on a supporting medium called the base, and is also subject to other coatings in order to protect it from damage. There are many ways of coating the base in order to produce a film with particular characteristics, but in order not to unduly confuse the discussion on the emulsion, the specifics of commonly available film types are considered in the next section (see Basic film types, p. 52). It is perhaps surprising to note that even with advances in computerised data storage techniques, film emulsion is still the most common way to provide 'hard copy' for the radiologist or physician.

Silver halides

Many light-sensitive materials are known, but very few possess the characteristics necessary for use in a photographic emulsion. The principal materials in use are the silver halides, metallic crystalline solids formed by reacting a suitable silver compound with one of the group of elements known as the halogens. There are four halogens, but only three produce a combination with silver that is useful in the photographic emulsions. These are:

- Silver bromide (AgBr)
- Silver iodide (AgI)
- Silver chloride (AgCl).

All three have a natural spectral sensitivity that ends in the 'blue' part of the visible spectrum at approximately 480 nm, i.e. they are not sensitive to light with wavelengths longer than about 480 nm. Also, the pure form of each of the three halides is of no use photographically, as they are all unable to form a usable latent image (see Ch. 6, Photochemistry). It is only the presence of the gelatine and other impurities deliberately added during manufacture which introduce imperfections to the crystal structure and enable a useful image to form.

Silver bromide (AgBr)

Silver bromide is the most used silver halide in emulsion manufacture. When used on its own it has a 'cut-off' sensitivity of approximately 480 nm and a 'peak' sensitivity at approximately 430 nm. The cut-off sensitivity is the wavelength above which the film is not sensitive, while the peak sensitivity is the wavelength to which the film is most sensitive (Fig. 4.4).

Practical emulsions are rarely pure silver bromide (with some notable exceptions, see tabular grains, p. 46) but are usually mixed with a small percentage of silver iodide. This small amount, of the order of 2–4%, has the effect of increasing the speed of the emulsion (i.e. its sensitivity) and altering its spectral sensitivity. Figure 4.5 shows the relevant spectrogram. The mixing of the silver iodide and bromide should mean that we refer to these emulsions as iodobromide emulsions; however, as the proportion of silver iodide is so low, common usage has resulted in X-ray emulsions being termed silver bromide only. It should be noted that a mix of two halides produces grains

that contain both halides in the same structure but not in the same proportion in all grains, i.e. not separate grains of the individual halides.

Silver chloride (AgCl)

Silver chloride has a low inherent sensitivity when compared to silver bromide and this disadvantage precludes its use in X-ray-type emulsions. It has, however, an advantage for certain applications in that it possesses very rapid development and fixing properties.

Silver iodide (AgI)

Silver iodide is only used in combination with either silver bromide or silver chloride. When used in combination with silver bromide it increases its sensitivity and marginally extends its spectral response (see Figs 4.4, 4.5). It is the effect that AgI has on speed that makes it particularly useful in

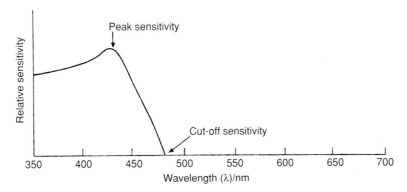

Fig. 4.4 Spectrogram showing the sensitivity of silver bromide (AgBr).

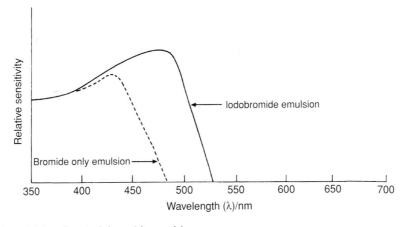

Fig. 4.5 Spectral sensitivity of an iodobromide emulsion.

X-ray emulsions. Unfortunately AgI has two important disadvantages:

- First, the presence of iodide in the emulsion significantly extends the time taken for the film to fix

- Second, it possesses certain chemical characteristics, irrelevant here, which preclude its use without either silver bromide or silver chloride.

However, having said that, the increase in fixing time is of little practical significance since most automatic processors adequately fix the film in approximately 22 seconds.

SPECTRAL SENSITIVITY

The spectral sensitivity of the emulsion is the range of wavelengths of the electromagnetic spectrum to which the emulsion will respond. Alternatively, it may be considered as the range of wavelengths that the emulsion will record as a latent image (whether that latent image is useful or not is irrelevant). Response of an emulsion is usually represented graphically by a spectrogram. It is a plot of a suitable measure of sensitivity against wavelength expressed as nanometers (Fig. 4.6).

The sensitivity measure may range from something as vague as relative sensitivity to something as explicit as log X,

$$\text{where } X = \left[\frac{\mu J}{cm^2}\right]$$

There seems to be no standard starting point for the wavelength scale and it appears to be chosen to suit the emulsion being illustrated. However, most films used in radiology use a starting point of 300 nm. Other significant parts of the spectrogram are *peak sensitivity* and *cut-off sensitivity*.

Peak sensitivity. Peak sensitivity is the wavelength or range of wavelengths at which the emulsion exhibits its highest response, i.e. the wavelength to which it is most sensitive.

Cut-off sensitivity. Cut-off sensitivity is the wavelength beyond which the film is no longer sensitive.

The spectral sensitivity of film emulsions can be conveniently divided into three sections:

- Monochromatic emulsions
- Orthochromatic emulsions
- Panchromatic emulsions.

Each of these divisions describes the range of wavelengths to which the emulsion will respond. Before considering each in detail we must first take a brief look at the generalities.

SPECTRAL SENSITISING

When used on their own, silver bromide emulsions have their cut-off sensitivity at approximately 480 nm. This is only marginally improved by adding silver iodide (see Figs 4.4, 4.5). In simple terms this means that silver bromide is sensitive only to blue light, the other colours of the spec-

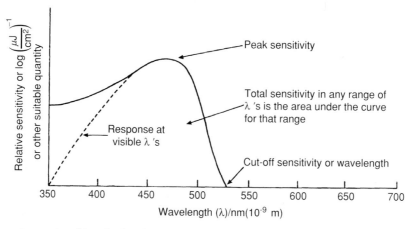

Fig. 4.6 Typical spectrogram and 'cardinal' points.

trum making no contribution to image production. In practice this limitation of an emulsion's ability to respond only to a small range of visible wavelengths has certain advantages and disadvantages, for example:

- Limiting the spectral sensitivity of a film allows it to be handled using suitable safelights and therefore makes processing and loading the film into cassettes much easier

- It limits the amount of information the film may record, but again this depends on the 'spectral nature' of the 'object' that film is exposed to.

A general rule that seems to hold true is that the film should be able to record the whole of the spectral output of the object it is trying to image.

Extending the natural sensitivity of the silver halides is achieved by adding a suitable dye to the emulsion. This principle was discovered in 1873 by Vogel, who managed to extend spectral sensitivity into the green part of the spectrum. Other dyes, which extended spectral response into the red and infrared, followed. The use of dyes in this way is termed:

- Spectral sensitising
- Dye sensitising
- Colour sensitising

or

- Optical sensitising.

Dyes that can achieve this feat are called colour sensitisers. The use of the word 'dye' is not an accident, as the materials used are literally coloured dyes. These dyes are added to the emulsion during manufacture and are designed to cover the surface of the silver bromide crystal. The amount of dye required is very small, of the order of only one molecule thick over the whole surface of the grain. This 'monolayer' may occasionally be extended to three or more molecules thick in exceptional circumstances.

Unsensitised emulsion. The silver bromide crystal has the ability to absorb all wavelengths up to 480 nm (blue). This absorption then releases free electrons into the crystal structure forming the latent image (see Ch. 6, Photochemistry), and longer wavelengths pass through the crystal with no effect.

Sensitised emulsion. The layer of dye surrounding the crystal allows the shorter 'blue' wavelengths into the crystal but absorbs, say, the longer 'green' wavelengths and converts these into electrons which then contribute to latent image formation.

Note that:

- Absorption of wavelengths longer than about 480 nm is achieved at the surface of the crystal by the use of dyes in layers that may be only one molecule thick

- The sensitivity of a 'dyed' emulsion is always *additional* to the parent crystal's inherent sensitivity

- It is important not to confuse spectral sensitising with the production of a 'coloured picture'.

This section has been concerned with a monochrome (i.e. black and white) material's ability to detect colour changes in a subject and register these changes as an alteration in shades of grey, *not* in the production of a true 'colour image' which is a complex topic beyond the scope of this book.

MONOCHROMATIC EMULSIONS

Monochromatic emulsions are variously known as blue sensitive, non-colour sensitive or blind emulsions, as well as other variations of these terms. 'Blind' is a term often used by manufacturers, as the emulsion cannot 'see' any colours of longer wavelength than blue. Figure 4.7 is a typical spectrogram for a monochromatic screen-type X-ray film. These emulsions are generally composed of globular grains (see Grain technology, p. 45) and are particularly useful in calcium tungstate, blue-emitting rare earth and ultraviolet-emitting screens systems. Their use in ultraviolet screens is particularly marked due to the low degree of crossover produced when using these systems. (For references on screens, see Ch. 5.)

ORTHOCHROMATIC EMULSIONS

Orthochromatic emulsions are those emulsions that have a spectral sensitivity up to and including the 'green' part of the visible spectrum.

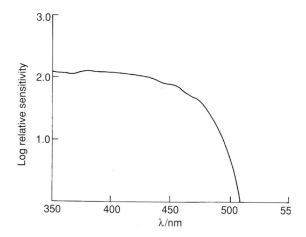

Fig. 4.7 Spectrogram of typical monochromatic screen-type X-ray emulsion.

The term orthochromatic is in fact a misnomer, as literally it means 'correct colour' and was used by the developers of these emulsions as they believed they had an emulsion sensitive to all the spectrum.

The extension of the spectral response, as compared to monochromatic emulsions, is achieved by spectral sensitising, using dye sensitising agents. These dyes allow the green parts of the visible spectrum to be absorbed at the surface of the silver halide grain and thus contribute to image formation (see also Spectral sensitising, p. 42, and Grain technology, p. 45).

Up to now the discussion has been rather vague, using the term 'green part of the visible spectrum'. This has been deliberate, as modern orthochromatic emulsions can be subdivided into the following:

- Short orthochromatic
- Medium orthochromatic
- Long orthochromatic.

The three are differentiated by the exact position of their spectral cut-off sensitivity, and peak sensitivity is achieved by careful selection of the sensitising dye. In turn this governs the portion of the 'green' part of the spectrum that will be absorbed. Figure 4.8 is a spectrogram illustrating typical responses of short, medium and long orthochromatic emulsions. These are not of particular film types but illustrate general principles. Details of particular films are available from manufacturers.

Uses of film with orthochromatic characteristics are numerous, for example green-emitting rare earth screens, monitor photography, photofluorography, certain cine films, etc. Its use is indicated whenever the 'object' to be imaged contains a high proportion of light from the green part of the visible spectrum.

PANCHROMATIC EMULSIONS

Panchromatic materials have a spectral sensitivity that covers all the wavelengths of the visible spectrum. Again, as with orthochromatic materials, they are sensitised to wavelengths longer

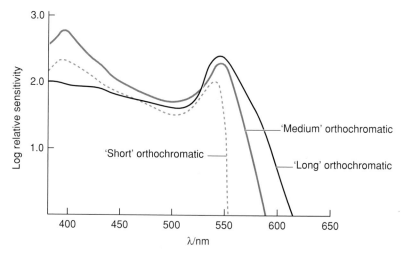

Fig. 4.8 Spectrogram showing examples of short, medium and long orthochromatic emulsions.

than blue light by the use of dye sensitising agents.

The use of these materials in radiography has been limited by the fact that they are not particularly 'user friendly', in that they must be handled in complete darkness until processed. Additionally there is no particular advantage from a technical point of view, as most present imaging techniques would benefit little from the use of these emulsions. Figure 4.9 is a typical spectrogram of a panchromatic material. Most of these films are differentiated by variations in the position of their long wave cut-off sensitivity.

For the sake of completeness, it must be mentioned that spectral sensitivity can be extended into the infrared part of the spectrum, to approximately 1200 nm. These materials are of particular use in aerial photography, scientific and technical photography, medical photography and the production of special effects. Technical difficulties encountered in the use of these films negate their common use.

GRAIN TECHNOLOGY

The subject of grain technology has assumed significant importance in recent times, especially with the move towards the greater use of orthochromatic-type emulsions in general radiography.

As far as radiography is concerned, we can divide grain technology into two sections:

- Globular grains
- Tabular grains.

Globular grains

In blue sensitive or monochromatic systems, globular grains are always used. This is because in the wavelengths up to blue, the light-absorbing ability of the grain depends only on its volume. If the emulsion needs to have a higher speed, i.e. an increased sensitivity, then research shows that the silver bromide grains should be a compact spherical shape, hence the name globular (Fig. 4.10). The spherical shape provides:

- High volume
- Good absorption

without excessive unsharpness in relation to film speed. The surface area of the grain has no effect on the amount of light absorbed.

If it is necessary to extend the spectral sensitivity of a globular grain into the green or red part of the visible spectrum, then a dye sensitising agent must be used. This is a layer of coloured dye that is absorbed into the surface of the silver bromide crystal. It may be up to a maximum of three molecules thick, but normally a monolayer is sufficient. The dye absorbs light of wavelengths longer than blue and releases the absorbed photons as electrons that can contribute to image formation. The extension of the spectral sensitivity in this way depends on the colour of the dye and is a 'surface' phenomenon,

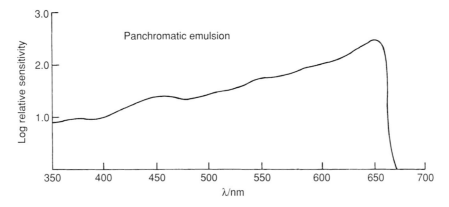

Fig. 4.9 Spectrogram showing typical panchromatic emulsion.

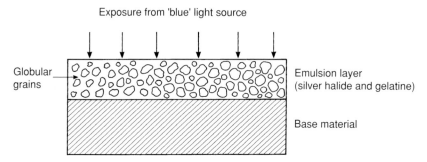

Fig. 4.10   Diagrammatic representation of globular grains.

i.e. the dye sensitising agent is absorbed at the surface of the grain and the wavelengths longer than blue are absorbed by the dye and therefore also at the surface. It is apparent that the ideal grain to maximise this effect would be one of little or no volume but which would present maximum surface area to the incoming light photons and therefore enhance absorption.

Tabular grains

These are grains of a particular shape that are used exclusively in sensitised emulsions. In radiography, orthochromatic sensitising of tabular grains is used in screen film technology. These grains can be divided into two main types:

- T-Mat emulsions
- Structured Twin emulsions.

Tabular grains have a 'table top'-like structure (Fig. 4.11), which provides a very large surface area but has a small volume. They are therefore particularly suitable for sensitisation as they present a large surface area to the dye and increase the amount of absorption possible.

Tabular grains are not particularly new; they have been known since about 1963, and have been used in high resolution colour films for many years. They are particularly impressive in that they produce a high speed emulsion with very high resolution and relatively low silver coating weights.

T-Mat™ emulsions

T-Mat is a registered trademark of Kodak Limited, who were first to introduce this form of technology into X-ray-type emulsions. A T-Mat™ emulsion is a tabular grain emulsion of a specific type (Fig. 4.12). In a conventional tabular grain emulsion there is always a small proportion of grains that are not flat. T-Mat™ technology makes an emulsion in which nearly all the grains are identical and extremely flat. The patent for T-Mat™ then goes on to specify surface diameter/thickness ratios for the individual silver bromide grains. Interestingly, these are silver bromide only emulsions and this situation somewhat limits the ability of the crystal to absorb the dye sensitising agent.

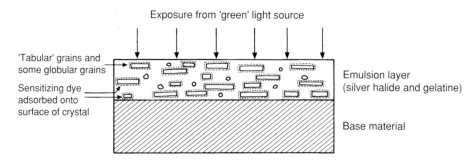

Fig. 4.11   Diagrammatic representation of tabular grains.

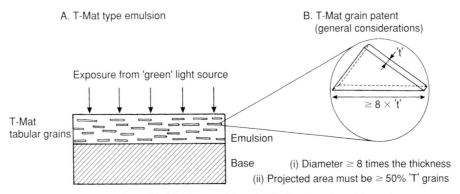

Fig. 4.12 Diagrammatic representation of (A) T-Mat emulsion; (B) T-Mat silver bromide grain.

There are some distinct advantages to this technology, particularly in the area of sharpness. The gain in sharpness is primarily due to a decrease in the amount of crossover, which can be as high as 75% in orthochromatic emulsions, to about 37%. This is simply because the flatter grains have a greater capacity to absorb light than spherical grains (Fig. 4.13). However, the gain in sharpness produces a marked increase in 'graininess' which is very easily visible.

Note that crossover is a feature of duplitised emulsions in which light from one screen exposes not only the emulsion closest to it but passes through the base and exposes the emulsion furthest away (see Ch. 5, Intensifying screens).

Structured Twin™ emulsions

ST or Structured Twin is a trademark of Agfa-Gevaert Limited. As with T-Mat™, it is a form of tabular grain technology, but in this case the increase in the surface area of the crystal is achieved by using two tabular-type grains in combination, hence the name 'Structured Twin'. Close examination of the exact crystal structure of T and ST™ grains will reveal major differences between the two. However, both technologies have the same approach, producing a crystal that has a large surface area compared to its volume, and conferring sensitivity by dye sensitisation. ST™ grains are more 'conventional', being a mix of silver bromide and iodide, and this improves the ability of the crystal to absorb more dye into its surface.

Again, the main advantage is to improve sharpness by reducing crossover. Figure 4.14 is a diagrammatic representation of a Structured Twin-type grain and a conventional T grain.

Advantages of tabular grains

The advantages of tabular grains are potentially significant. However, in order to realise some of

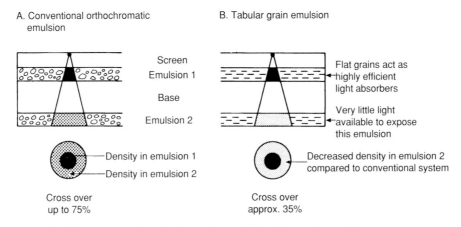

Fig. 4.13 Crossover in (A) conventional orthochromatic and (B) tabular grain emulsions.

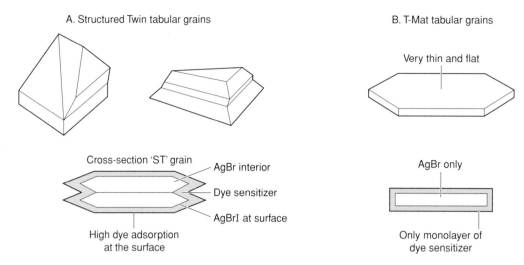

A. Structured Twin tabular grains

B. T-Mat tabular grains

Very thin and flat

Cross-section 'ST' grain

AgBr interior

Dye sensitizer

AgBrI at surface

High dye adsorption
at the surface

AgBr only

Only monolayer of
dye sensitizer

Fig. 4.14   Diagrammatic representation of (A) Structured Twin tabular grains; (B) T-Mat tabular grains.

these advantages a radical rethink of attitudes towards films and processing would be required. The following is a list of some of the possible advantages. Only a few are immediately available, and only some will find their way into the imaging department:

- Increased resolution when compared to a film of conventional grain technology with the same speed; this is mainly due to reduction in crossover.

- Reduction in silver coating weights: making the crystals thinner and flatter reduces the amount of silver used in manufacture. This does not affect sensitivity, as green light absorption now takes place in the dye layer at the surface of the crystal. Blue light is absorbed in the volume of the crystal, but this is almost irrelevant when using green-emitting rare earth screens.

- Theoretically suitable for 45 s processing; this is mainly due to the reduction in silver coating weights, coupled with the fact that it is easier to harden the film (in fact it may be possible to totally harden the film in manufacture) and the fact that it simplifies developer chemistry.

Disadvantage of tabular grains

- Higher graininess; this is mainly due to the better imaging of quantum mottle, rather than

to an increase in true film grain. Almost entirely due to the reduction in crossover.

Other grain technology

Many manufacturers are using other kinds of grain technology; a detailed discussion of these would fill a book in its own right. In an attempt to illustrate this, the following is a list of high resolution films and the particular grain technology used:

- SMG grains: surface modified grains (Fuji)
- CLG grains: concentrated latent image grains (Fuji)
- HMG grains: high ortho mono-dispersed grains (Konica).

This is not intended to be a complete list, but illustrates the efforts being made to advance grain technology.

Grain size and distribution

Grain size and distribution are governed during manufacture when the emulsion is undergoing the first ripening stage of production. Here the crystals grow to the required size, correct distribution is achieved and this fixes the emulsion speed, contrast and graininess characteristics.

In the not-too-distant past it was possible to be quite specific as to what effects grain size and distribution would have on contrast and speed. However, with the advent of the dye sensitised tabular-type grains this delineation into separate groupings has become less relevant. The good news is that the generalities still apply, especially when considering globular grain emulsion.

Contrast

The degree of contrast produced depends on grain size distribution, i.e. the range of grain sizes. An emulsion that has a wide range of grain sizes produces a film that has a low film contrast. This is because the film is sensitive to a wide range of exposures and therefore has high exposure latitude and, by the rules of sensitometry, must have low film contrast. At a crystalline level this is because the larger crystals are most sensitive and the smaller crystals least sensitive to exposure. The sensitivity of intermediate sizes varies accordingly. Therefore a wide range of grain sizes implies a wide sensitivity to exposure and, because of the above argument, a low contrast film. It follows that a small range of grain sizes produces a film with high contrast and, in the limit, a film with only one grain size produces virtually no grey scale but very high contrast.

In practice the production of emulsions with a narrow range of grain sizes is quite difficult and these films are useful only in highly specialised situations.

Speed

The speed of an emulsion is governed by its average grain size. In general, the larger the average grain size, the more sensitive the film and the greater its speed. The reverse is also true. With dye sensitised emulsions this general rule is somewhat more complicated. Consider two emulsions, both with the same average grain size and general crystal shape. If one emulsion is monochromatic and the other orthochromatic in its spectral response and both are exposed to a light source containing the whole of the visible spectrum, then the orthochromatic film will apparently have a higher speed. This is simply because it is capable of recording more of the wavelengths of the light exposing it as an image. These features open up some interesting possibilities; for example, an orthochromatic film can have a lower silver coating weight than its monochromatic alternative and still have the same speed class (assuming the correct screens are used), or a smaller average grain size but again the same speed class. It must be remembered, however, that other factors may become more relevant, in terms of the final image quality, as radiographic systems become more complex.

Finally, the production of high speed emulsions with large grain sizes usually results in the simultaneous growth of other grains of smaller sizes. Inevitably this means that fast film tends towards low contrast and slower film towards high contrast.

Graininess

The subject of graininess is a complex topic which comprises many variables. As far as the film emulsion is concerned, the silver halide crystals are responsible for what is called 'true film grain'. True film grain is not visible to the naked eye; even the largest crystals are very small, being only about 1 micron in diameter ($1\mu = 10^{-6}$ m). However, a grainy pattern can usually be detected with little or no magnification. This is owing to the fact that the grains are spatially distributed not only in area but also in depth, giving the appearance of being clumped together and forming random density variations in areas that should appear as an homogeneous density. Grains may also be actually clumped together (i.e. in physical contact) as a result of techniques of manufacture or processing.

The rule of thumb usually applied to film grain is to say that the faster the film, the larger the grains and the greater the degree of graininess. In practice this proves to be quite accurate, but certainly as far as film and screen combinations are concerned, by far the largest contributing factor to graininess is quantum mottle. (A more complete insight into graininess is given in Ch. 9, Image quality.)

GELATINE

Gelatine is a complex common protein deriving its name from the Latin *gelata* ('formation in water'). The common misconception is that it is produced from horses' hooves, muscle tissue or blood. It is not. Commercial manufacture is based on white fibrous connective tissue, or more correctly collagen fibres, the principal sources of which are cartilage, skin and ossein (the protein matrix of bone).

Collagen is converted into gelatine by the process known as hydrolysis (which is the chemical decomposition of a substance by water). During this conversion the water destroys the crosslinking of the collagen, and this produces the gelatine polymer (Fig. 4.15).

No definite structure or size has been determined for the gelatine molecule since it is a mixture of degradation products. However, its general form is thought to be:

$$(NH_2CH_2COOH)_n$$

Commercial manufacture

Figure 4.16 is an abbreviated flow diagram of the various stages involved in the manufacture of gelatine. Photographically, it is the curing process that has the first important effect on the nature of the emulsion. It is here that the *isoelectric point* of the emulsion is determined and this has profound consequences on the film's final characteristics.

Isoelectric point (IEP)

The isoelectric point of an emulsion is very significant in determining certain important characteristics. It depends on the type of gelatine and is

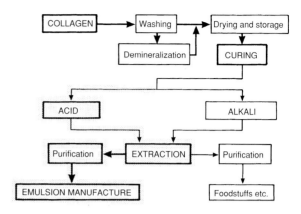

Fig. 4.16 The manufacture of gelatine.

defined as 'the pH value at which a substance or system is electrically neutral'.

Acid cure gelatine has a low isoelectric point, being electrically neutral at a typical value of pH 4.85, while alkali cure has a high isoelectric point at approximately 7.8 pH (Fig. 4.17). From a photographic point of view, the isoelectric point effectively:

- Determines how easily products are removed from the emulsion
- Affects the degree of hardening.

At its isoelectric point, gelatine has the following properties:

- Minimum solubility
- Minimum viscosity
- Minimum conductivity
- Minimum swelling.

The isoelectric point can be altered by the addition of suitable contaminants, thus allowing fine control of the factors listed above. Emulsions can therefore have a variable range of properties to suit very specialised applications.

One of the principal factors affecting the choice of an emulsion's IEP is the IEP of the by-products of processing that need to be removed. In general, if the by-products have a higher IEP than the emulsion, the products are easier to remove. In the case of conventional X-ray-type emulsions, an IEP of approximately 4.8 is usual as the majority of by-products requiring removal have IEPs greater than this value. It follows that gelatine used in the manufacture of these prod-

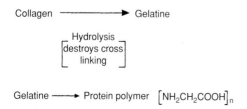

Fig. 4.15 The production of gelatine.

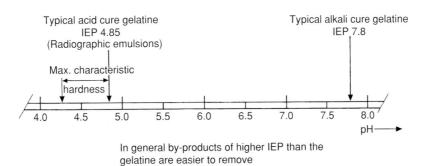

In general by-products of higher IEP than the gelatine are easier to remove

Fig. 4.17   Diagrammatic representation of isoelectric points (IEP).

ucts should be of the acid cure variety (see Fig. 4.17).

Finally, not only is the IEP of the emulsion significant, but the IEP of the supercoat (see p. 53) is also important. Medical X-ray films are conventionally low IEP emulsions with a low IEP supercoat due to the reasons outlined in the previous paragraph.

Function of gelatine

Photographically the function of gelatine can be divided into two sections:

- Physical properties
- Photographic properties.

Physical properties

Gelatine:

- Absorbs the water present in processing and can go from a sol to a gel and the reverse an infinite number of times. In the act of changing from a sol to a gel the gelatine swells, opens its molecular structure, and allows easy penetration of processing solutions.

- Keeps the silver bromide in suspension and assists in keeping the individual crystals separate from each other. This reduces the amount of grain clumping.

- Binds the emulsion to the film base. A thin layer of pure material is often included as part of the manufacturing process to literally 'glue' the emulsion to the base (see Substratum, p. 53).

- Provides a growth medium during emulsion manufacture allowing the silver halide crystals to develop to the required size.

Photographic properties

- Gelatine provides impurities of sulphur which give active points of silver sulphide (Ag_2S) within the crystal structure. These points deepen electron traps and consume certain photo by-products (see Latent image formation, p. 91). The amount of impurity added is carefully controlled during manufacture in order to produce an emulsion with the desired characteristics.

- Gelatine allows and encourages the production of electron traps due to the formation of crystal defects. Electron traps are vital during the formation of the latent image and without them there would be no photography as we know it (see Latent image formation, p. 91).

- During exposure some of the silver bromide is split into its component ions ($Ag^+ + Br^-$). Gelatine helps prevent the recombination of the bromine ions after their release by exposure.

- Gelatine reduces the rate of the back reaction and prevents the effects of exposure becoming undone; i.e. it reduces latent image fade.

Age fog

The advantage of gelatine providing sulphur impurities also has a disadvantage in that it increases the amount of fog formed on unexposed film, even if all storage factors are ideal.

Age fog is due to the increase in the amount of silver sulphide in the emulsion with storage. This increase renders the silver bromide crystal more susceptible to development. Some silver sulphide is 'built in' to the crystal so it is suitable for latent image formation; the rest comes from the colloidal sulphur (present in the emulsion gelatine) combining with either free interstitial silver ions or actual crystal lattice ions.

BASIC FILM TYPES

There is a wide variety of film types available to suit many different needs, ranging from those of the astronomer to those of the amateur photographer. In radiography there is still a significant choice of film types but the basic structures of the films found in imaging departments fall into three basic categories:

- Duplitised
- Single-coated
- Double-coated.

The specifics of each type will be discussed in some detail in the sections that follow. However, it is sufficient to say now that duplitised films have the emulsion layer on both sides of the film base, single-coated films have an emulsion layer on only one side of the film base, and double-coated films have two emulsion layers but both are on the same side of the film base (in this case they are usually different emulsion types). Triple-coated films do exist, the best example of these being conventional colour print and slide films typically used in 35 mm cameras.

DUPLITISED FILMS

These are films with emulsion coated on both sides of the film base. The general structure and typical dimensions are shown in Figure 4.18. This represents a screen-type film. As the figure shows, it is composed of various layers, each with a particular function.

The base

The base acts as a supporting medium for the other layers and may be one of several materials, such as glass, cellulose triacetate or paper. However, *all* X-ray films are coated on a 'polyester base' (or, to be more technically accurate, polyethylene teraphthalate). Polyester has many advantages that encourage its use:

- Dimensional stability
- Optical clarity
- Waterproof
- High tensile strength
- Flexible
- Chemical 'memory'
- Inert to processing chemicals
- Conforms to non-flammability regulations (i.e. is a safety base).

All these factors combine to produce a material that is particularly suitable for automatic roller processing at high temperatures; indeed, it was the introduction of polyester base that cured many of the problems associated with early roller processors.

The base can either be coloured or clear. It should be appreciated that the choice of colour for the base material is not arbitrary, but has a sound scientific basis.

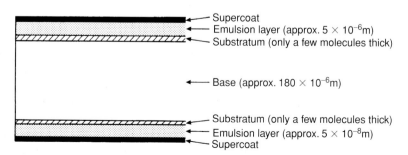

Supercoat
Emulsion layer (approx. 5×10^{-6}m)
Substratum (only a few molecules thick)

Base (approx. 180×10^{-6}m)

Substratum (only a few molecules thick)
Emulsion layer (approx. 5×10^{-8}m)
Supercoat

Fig. 4.18 Duplitised film: cross-sectional structure and dimensions.

Blue base. The choice of a blue-based film can give some distinct benefits:

- In continuous viewing, blue-based material is much more restful on the viewer's eyes

- Blue-based material also produces a slightly higher visual contrast than clear base

- In general, a blue base gives a more aesthetically pleasing image. Although this is obviously subjective, large numbers of people choose a blue-based material in preference to clear base.

However, one disadvantage of blue base is that if it is viewed on a poor quality, yellow-light emitting viewing box, the film will have an apparent high base fog.

Clear base. In contrast:

- Clear base has a very low base fog when compared to a blue-based film. This is due to the fact that density is contributed by the base *only* and it is usually extremely low.

- The basic fog of clear-based film remains low even when viewed on poor viewing equipment. There is also a slight increase in perceptibility in the toe of the curve due to the lower base fog, which makes this type of base particularly suitable for ultrasound work.

Clear base does, however, produce slightly lower visual contrast.

Continued viewing of a clear-based film may be more tiresome for some viewers.

Substratum

Also known as the subbing layer, this is an adhesive layer that literally sticks the emulsion to the base. The choice of substance for this function primarily depends on the nature of the base material. If the base is of the acetate type, then it is a very thin, almost monolayer of gelatine; however, polyester base is not so easy and poses some considerable problems.

The single main problem is finding a material that has adhesive qualities and also an affinity for both the natural gelatine organic polymer and the man-made 'polyester' polymer. In the early days of polyester base this was somewhat

problematic, but the problems were soon overcome by rapid advances in technology.

Emulsion

The specific details of the film's emulsion have been fully considered earlier in this chapter. It is sufficient to state here that the emulsion is a mixture of gelatine and one of, or a mixture of, the silver halides of bromine, chlorine and iodine.

The shapes of the crystals in this suspension may range from globular to tabular grains, according to the use the emulsion will be put to, and there may be dye sensitising agents present in order to control the spectral sensitivity characteristics of the film. X-ray films are principally silver bromide emulsions.

Supercoat

This is a thin layer of clear, specially hardened gelatine that is coated onto the top surface of the emulsion. Its purpose is to protect the emulsion from mechanical damage and provide the required surface characteristics.

The most usual mechanical damage is abrasion marks due to roller transportation in processing and mishandling; this is minimised by making the supercoat as smooth and as hard as possible. However, it must not be too smooth, as a certain amount of 'roughness' is required to enable the film to transport through roller processors and automated film-handling systems. Likewise it must not be too hard, as this could make the penetration of the processing chemistry more difficult and extend processing times. A suitable compromise is therefore made between all significant factors.

Screen-type duplitised films

With all the information available from manufacturers it seems, at first, that numerous different film types are available. Closer examination reveals that, in the case of screen-type duplitised films, availability can conveniently be divided into three sections, with only subtle variations in basic characteristics between different manufacturers' products within each section:

1. 'Conventional' or standard contrast-type
2. Half speed-type
3. 'Latitude'-type.

Each type may be available in either monochromatic or orthochromatic spectral sensitivities (depending on the screen type with which it is to be used; see Ch. 5, Intensifying screens), as well as conventional or advanced technology grain emulsions. The variation in characteristics between each of the divisions provides the facility to choose the best possible combination of film and screen to enable an image of the highest possible diagnostic content to be produced, with regard to other significant factors such as dose, etc. The advantage to the patient is obvious.

'Standard contrast'-type emulsions

Conventional or standard contrast-type emulsions are so called for historical reasons: films with these general contrast characteristics were originally the most often used. It is comparison with this type that has resulted in the names of the other two, i.e. half speed and 'L'.

The features of conventional emulsions are best considered by examining their sensitometric characteristics (Fig. 4.19), and then comparing the other two types to this base line. To ensure that the comparison is fair, it is assumed that each film is exposed to a light source of spectral emission that corresponds to the film's sensitivity, that the same source is used in each case, and that each film receives identical processing.

Figure 4.19 shows a typical characteristic curve for a standard contrast-type emulsion:

- Base + fog = 0.18;
- Average gradient ($\bar{G}$) = 2.6
- Maximum density (D max) = 3.5–4.0, and
- Speed = log It 1.53 (at net density 1.0).

These values are not representative of any specific emulsion, but illustrate the general case.

Half speed-type emulsions

As the name implies, these films have approximately half the speed of their conventional counterparts. The reduction in speed generally improves the image quality but increases the dose to the patient. However, the use of half speed film with high speed rare earth screens to produce a certain 'speed class' (i.e. the speed of film and screen in combination) seems to produce improved image quality when compared to a 'conventional' film and screens in the same speed class. The use of such a film greatly increases the range of film/screen combinations available to suit dif-

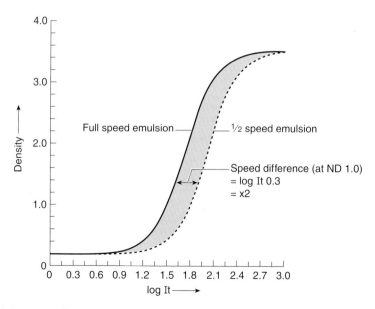

Fig. 4.19 Characteristic curves of conventional and 'half speed'-type emulsions.

fering situations. Unfortunately, making the choice of which combination to use is not simple.

The reduction in speed is achieved by reducing the silver coating weight of the emulsion (although it is not reduced by one-half, as the relationship between speed and coating weight is not that simple). Again, Figure 4.19 shows the essential characteristics. All factors are similar except the speed, which is decreased to log It 1.83.

Finally, it is as well to note that half speed emulsions are available in standard contrast and/or latitude ('L')-type emulsion coatings.

Latitude or 'L'-type emulsions

These emulsions were specifically introduced to improve the detail seen in the peripheral areas of the chest radiography. With standard contrast emulsions, detail tends to be lost in these areas as they are at the upper limit of the useful density range, and of high subject contrast due to the air acting as a negative contrast agent.

In an 'L'-type emulsion, the silver halide grain size distribution within a particular size range is so arranged that, at higher densities, the gradient of the characteristic curve decreases. This decreases the subject contrast enhancement and increases the latitude (i.e. increases grey scale) in high density areas (Fig. 4.20). Thus a film of high perceptibility in both high and low density areas can be made.

When applied to a chest radiograph, this means that the detail available should be similar over all the areas of the lung fields.

An obvious spin-off of this is that it also increases the film latitude and therefore the exposure latitude of the whole emulsion. Marketing of these film types has therefore concentrated on this wide latitude and the fact that this leads to fewer repeat examinations, especially in situations where exposure assessment is difficult (e.g. theatre). However, the visual appearance of this kind of emulsion is not to the liking of some radiologists and clinicians, and this emulsion has proved to be simply another addition to the types available.

Figure 4.20 is a typical characteristic curve of an 'L' emulsion. All the essential features are the same as for a standard contrast film (or half speed film, if that is being considered) except for the average gradient, which is reduced to $\bar{G} = 2.2$. The average gradient can be misleading here, as at lower densities the curve has a gradient similar to a conventional emulsion, whereas at higher densities it is somewhat less than the average (Fig. 4.20).

Resolution

Resolution values of screen-type emulsions are of no practical significance, as the limiting factor is not the film but the screen with which the film is being used. Therefore system resolution is

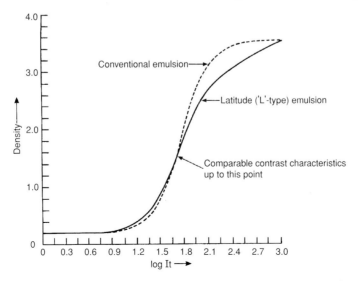

Fig. 4.20 Characteristic curve of a latitude ('L')-type emulsion (compared to a conventional emulsion).

used in preference. For a 200 class rare earth system with 'conventional' film, a typical value at 10% MTF would be six line pairs per millimetre (see Resolution, p. 169).

In general, within a speed class using the same film, rare earth screens have higher resolutions compared to calcium tungstate screens. Increasing speed class usually means decreasing resolution.

In all cases the resolution capabilities of the film greatly exceed that of the screens.

Reciprocity failure

This is a feature of very short exposure times at high intensities and very long times at low intensities not producing the density expected. It is always a problem when light is the principal image producer and therefore affects all film/screen systems.

In general it is not a problem if exposure times are kept between 0.003 s and 3 s. A fuller description of reciprocity failure is given in Chapter 5, Intensifying screens.

Advantages of duplitisation

Increased film speed

Doubling the amount of emulsion available to expose must increase the 'sensitivity' of the system. This is especially so when a duplitised film is used between a pair of intensifying screens.

For example, if a single screen with a single-coated film is exposed to an X-ray beam, about 10% of the beam will be converted into useful exposure on the film and 90% will be wasted. If another screen and emulsion are provided, a further 10% of that 90% can be made useful and contribute to the image; therefore, providing a second emulsion and screen approximately doubles the sensitivity of the system.

This increase in film speed has many advantages, the principal one being that it reduces:

- Dose to the patient
- Movement unsharpness (due to decreased exposure times)
- Geometric unsharpness (e.g. if smaller focal spots are used)
- Potential dose to staff.

Increased contrast

In simple terms, contrast is the difference in density between two adjacent areas on the film. A duplitised film will always have the potential to have higher contrast than single-coated film of the same coating weight because higher density differences are possible with the same exposure owing to the presence of a higher level of available density-producing silver halide. Thus density differences are always potentially greater from duplitised than from single-coated materials.

Disadvantages of duplitisation

The largest single disadvantage of duplitisation is the increase in photographic unsharpness due to the parallax effect. Consider the build-up of an image of a narrow slit in the emulsion (Fig. 4.21). When viewed perpendicular to the plane of the film, the images are perfectly superimposed and appear as one. However, because the two images are spatially separated, if they are viewed at an angle the edges of the image will appear unsharp as the two images are slightly displaced from each other – i.e. they look 'blurred'. The effect of this blurring is very limited as the distances between the emulsion layers are very small, and in any case other unsharpness factors are more significant.

Under certain conditions, though, it can become a problem, for example, in the days of manual processing, films were often viewed in their 'wet' state and a provisional diagnosis made. This was always followed up by a report when the films were dry, due to the fact that the parallax unsharpness caused by the wet swollen emulsion was unacceptable.

Other duplitised emulsions

In any attempt to generalise it is inevitable that certain items will not conveniently fit into the proposed categories. It is the same in this case. The following film emulsions, which are included in an attempt to be as comprehensive as possible, are available, but are not in such common use as the ones described above.

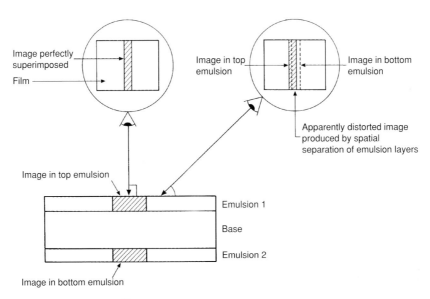

Fig. 4.21 Image distortion due to parallax.

Split emulsion films

These films are designed specifically for mammography. Each layer is formed by mono-dispersed cubic crystals. A cross-section taken through the film will demonstrate the following layers:

- Protective top coating
- Cubic crystal emulsion layer 1
- Cubic crystal emulsion layer 2
- Base
- Anti-halation layer
- Protective top coating.

Emulsion layer 1 is designed to provide high contrast, and layer 2 to give a high D max and contrast. The mono-dispersed cubic crystal technology is formed by grains which are identical in size, thus reducing the image graininess. The latent image is formed on the edge of the crystal resulting in a faster processing time being required.

Contrast or 'C' type emulsions

This type is very popular with certain physicians, particularly in the USA. It is a *very* low contrast mono- or orthochromatic emulsion with fog and speed characteristics similar to standard contrast films. Particularly designed for chest radiography, it has wide grey scale rendition that makes the film appear to be lacking in detail, especially to the untrained observer. Again the subjective choice of the radiologist or clinician is of great importance.

High speed emulsions

As the name suggests, these are high speed films. They produce (approximately) an 800 speed class when used with regular screens (this would be 200 with standard speed films) and are advanced grain technology emulsions. This is necessary in order to maintain high resolution at high speeds, therefore they are orthochromatic in spectral sensitivity. All high speed tabular grain emulsions tend to have higher contrast than their conventional counterparts.

FILM FORMATS AND PACKAGING

Films are available in a vast array of sizes and different packaging to suit virtually all possible situations. In Europe, metric sizes are used almost exclusively, while imperial sizes still predominate in the USA. The following is a list of the most often-used metric sizes available from manufacturers:

18 × 24 cm
24 × 30 cm
30 × 40 cm
15 × 30 cm
35.5 × 35.5 cm
35.5 × 43 cm.

Packing

Film is usually supplied in boxes of 25, 50, 100 and 500 sheets and either NIF, FW or AFW wrapped (see below).

NIF stands for non-interleaved film. The film is not protected from its neighbours in any way, but scratch marks on the surface of the film are virtually non-existent. This is due to two factors; first, improved hardening of the supercoat protecting the film, and second the trend towards hermetically sealed vacuum/partial vacuum packs of foil or plastic. These packs hold the sheets of film firmly together in a single package, eliminating movement between adjacent sheets during transportation. Occasionally, severe mishandling can cause film movement and produce localised abrasion marks that appear as a 'bird's nest' of high density scratches. Not surprisingly, this is called transport abrasion, and is best seen using a magnifying glass after processing.

The film is further protected by placing the foil or plastic bag in a strong outer box of high quality card. Some manufacturers include a lead strip that completely encompasses the box or internal packing. This enables the user of the film to tell easily if it has accidentally been exposed to ionising radiation. The strip shows on the film as an area of low density below the general fog density on a film processed straight from the packet.

An additional advantage to hermetically sealed packaging is the fact that the relative humidity of the atmosphere during storage is less critical. The film is effectively enclosed in its own microclimate at the ideal moisture content to ensure maximum storage without an adverse effect on base + fog level – however, other factors may become more significant (see Ch. 8, Sensitometry).

FW stands for folder wrapped. In this packing each sheet of film is individually wrapped in a folded sheet of photographic quality paper. This is to reduce abrasion marks on the surface of the film, which may occur as the films rub against each other during transportation, removal from the film hopper and during loading into the cassette. Folder wrapping also acts as protection against finger marking.

AFW stands for alternate folder wrapped, i.e. every other film in the box has its own separate cover of paper. The paper used is one of the most pure that can be made and must be free of any contaminant that may adversely affect the emulsion. Particularly problematic is the presence of very low level radioactive material which, as it decays, 'exposes' the film, producing a mottled appearance after processing.

A particularly bad outbreak of 'paper mottle' occurred in the early 1970s in paper supplied from an originally pure source. It was eventually traced to very low level contamination in the water supply to a particular paper mill. Large amounts of film were affected, at some considerable cost to the manufacturers. Since this accident, manufacturers have tried to move towards NIF packing, with considerable success. This removes the chance of mottle and reduces packing costs.

Not every film size is available in FW or AFW, but most are sold in NIF packing. Film packed in 500s is a so-called 'econopack' and is usually subdivided into 4 × 125s within one large external pack. It is obviously most useful where a particular size has a high volume turnover, and normally has a cost advantage over smaller boxes (say 5 × 100) for the same amount.

DIRECT EXPOSURE DUPLITISED FILMS

The general structure of direct exposure film is the same as screen-type duplitised film (see Fig. 4.18). Films usually come in their own individual envelope with no need to reload into a cassette.

Differences between direct exposure and screen-type emulsions

- *Higher resolution.* In direct exposure emulsions, resolution is principally limited by average

AgBr grain size, unlike screen film in which it is limited by the particular screen in which the film is used.

- *Higher silver coating weight.* As the film is entirely dependent on X-rays or gamma rays for image production, it follows that density is built up by direct absorption of these rays by the AgBr in the emulsion. To increase the sensitivity of the emulsion, a higher silver coating weight is used; this increases the chance of the X-rays or gamma rays being absorbed. Typically, silver coating weights will be four times that of a screen film.

- *Lower speed.* When exposed in the conditions for which the film is designed their speed will be slower.

- *Higher maximum density.* Due to the fact that these emulsions have a higher silver weight, a higher maximum density is also possible. Typically this would be about density 6–7.

- *Higher contrast.* The average gradient of the characteristic curve measured between net density 1.5 and 3.5 would typically be a value of about 5.0, depending on processing, and represents a film with very high contrast when compared to a medical screen film ($\bar{G} = 2.5$ approximately).

The use of direct exposure films in medical radiography has declined in recent years due to the development of high resolution rare earth screen techniques which have the advantages of low patient dose and excellent image quality.

SINGLE-COATED EMULSIONS

Structure

The general structure of a single-coated film is shown in Figure 4.22. As can be seen, it has an emulsion layer on only one side of the base. The basic features of the structures on this side of the film are as previously discussed, although the emulsion layer will probably have a lower silver coating weight and be spectrally sensitised to wavelengths above 510 nm (blue), depending on its use. The non-emulsion side has some very significant features.

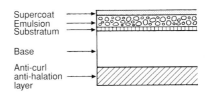

Fig. 4.22 Cross-section through a single-coated emulsion.

Anti-curl backing

This has the function, just as its name suggests, of preventing the film curling during processing and allows the film to stay flat after processing. Curling occurs as a result of the differential expansion of the emulsion caused by water absorption from the processing solutions. The base, however, is waterproof and dimensionally stable and therefore stays the same size. As the emulsion is attached to the base by the subbing layer, the film curls with the emulsion side out (somewhat similar in principle to a heated bi-metallic strip). To prevent this, another layer of gelatine is coated on the non-emulsion side. This expands to the same degree as the emulsion layer, equalising the stresses and ensuring that the film stays flat.

Halation

Halation, as shown in Figure 4.23, is caused by the reflection of light (which has already passed through the emulsion) at the boundary of the base with the air. If the angle of incidence is greater than the critical angle, the light may be reflected back and re-expose the emulsion layer. This produces a 'halo' unsharpness effect that reduces resolution. The density of the unsharp area is less than that of the true image.

Anti-halation layer

This is a coloured dye included in the gelatine of the anti-curl backing. In preventing *halation* it improves the resolution of the film:

- *Dyes used* in anti-halation layers are the subject of stringent patent protection by manufacturers, and are designed to absorb light that passes through the base and into the anti-curl/halation layer. Their principle of operation is based on the colour complimentary process which, in

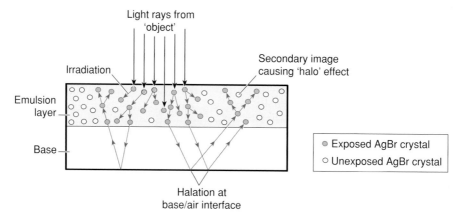

Fig. 4.23 Diagrammatic representation of halation and irradiation.

simple terms, means that if a certain colour light is passed through the correct colour filter, total absorption will take place and no light will pass through. In this context, therefore, halation cannot take place.

• *Dye removal*. The anti-halation dye must be removed in processing, otherwise correct viewing of the image is not possible (due to light absorption from the viewing box). This is achieved in the fixing bath and requires no special alteration to the chemistry. However, removal of the dye takes considerably more 'energy' out of the fixer than the exposed AgBr does, resulting in the need for higher fixer replenishment rates in processors that are using large volumes of single-coated emulsions.

Irradiation

This produces an effect similar to that of halation and is caused by the lateral scatter of light within the emulsion layer. The reflection makes developable AgBr crystals that are outside the true edge of the image, producing a 'halo'-type effect after processing. As this is produced within the emulsion layer, anti-halation backing will not prevent this effect (see Fig. 4.23).

Identification of emulsion side

In view of the factors considered in the previous section, it is vital to be able to determine accurately the emulsion side of the film. This is to ensure that it is loaded into the cassette the correct way round, so it faces the 'object' to be imaged, for example so it always faces the TV monitor in a multiformat camera, or the screen in a single screen mammographic technique.

Identification of the emulsion side is achieved by the manufacturer cutting a small notch out of the edge of the film. When this notch is positioned in the top right or bottom left corner, the emulsion is facing the person handling the film. Contrary to popular opinion, it is not possible to determine accurately the emulsion side by trying to judge which side is matt or shiny, or by 'tasting' the corner of the film.

FILMS FOR SPECIALISED USE

The general structural features of films to be found in the imaging department have already been discussed. Virtually all these films fall into the duplitised or single-coated emulsion categories. In the following section, specific details of film characteristics according to their use is presented. It should be noted that a full understanding of these details requires some knowledge of sensitometry; the reader is referred to Chapter 8.

Laser printing film

• *Use*. With imaging plates, and/or laser printers.

• *Film type*. Single-coated, fine grain emulsion with an anti-halation backing.

- *Spectral sensitivity*. Selected to match the type of laser being used.

- *Film formats*. 24 × 24 cm, 35 × 35 cm, 35 × 43 cm, 8 × 10 in, 10 × 12 in, 11 × 14 in.

- *Special features*. Available with either blue or clear base. Packaged for either darkroom or daylight processing. Can be used for ultrasound, CT, etc., or for conventional radiography with imaging plates.

Monitor photography

- *Use*. Imaging the video output from CT, MRI and ultrasound units and other similar modalities, usually via a multiformat or other camera system.

- *Film type*. Single-coated with anti-halo/curl backing.

- *Spectral sensitivity*. Short orthochromatic. Peak sensitivity in the order of 540 nm. Cut-off sensitivity in the order of 560 nm.

- *Film formats*. 5 in × 4 in up to 35 cm × 43 cm, to suit imaging camera in use.

- *Special features*. Available in blue or clear base and high or low contrast for use in ultrasound, etc.

Cine radiography

- *Use*. Cine recording of the output phosphor of a specialised image intensifier (usually in cardiography/cardiology departments).

- *Film type*. Single-coated.

- *Spectral sensitivity*. Long orthochromatic (see Fig. 4.8). Peak 550 nm. Cut-off in the order of 610 nm.

- *Film formats*. 35 mm × 90 m rolls emulsion coated inside, 35 mm × 180 m rolls emulsion coated inside or outside. Cut and perforated to DIN standard 15501; negative perforation short pitch, and conforms to ANSI P. H. 2293.

- *Special features*. Also suitable for other applications of intensifier photography and photofluorography. Stable reciprocity characteristics at exposures between 0.001 and 1.0 s.

Imaging intensifier photography and photofluorography

- *Use*. Recording the output phosphor of image intensifiers, especially those used for barium and associated techniques and mass miniradiography.

- *Film type*. Single-coated with anti-halo/anti-curl backing.

- *Spectral sensitivity*. Short orthochromatic (see Fig. 4.8). Peak sensitivity 540 nm. Cut-off sensitivity in the order of 570 nm.

- *Film formats*. Available as sheet film (100 × 100 mm) or roll film, 70 mm × 45 m; 90 mm × 30 m; 105 mm × 45 m.

- *Special features*. Variable contrast to suit individual radiologist choice and stable reciprocity characteristics between 0.001 and 1.0 s exposure.

Dental film

- *Use*. Intra-oral work.

- *Film type*. Direct exposure film, duplitised emulsion.

- *Spectral sensitivity*. As conventional film.

- *Film formats*. 5 × 7 cm, 3 × 4 cm, 2 × 3 cm.

- *Special features*. Covered in a 'waterproof' packet, and some manufacturers package two films together to enable two films to be produced from one exposure. There is a raised 'dot' on the film to denote the tube side after the film has been processed.

Copy or duplicating film

- *Use*. Producing exact copies in terms of size and density reproduction, by direct contact printing.

- *Film type*. Pre-solarised single-coated with anti-halo/anti-curl backing.

- *Spectral sensitivity*. Monochromatic but with peak sensitivity very much in the ultraviolet region of the spectrum, in the order of 350 nm.

- *Film formats*. Available as sheet film, usually in a whole range of sizes from 35 × 43 cm to 18 × 24 cm.

- *Special features*. A pre-solarised film is unusual in that an increase in exposure received results in a decrease in density. The average gradient should be as close to 1 as possible, to ensure accurate reproduction of the 'object film's' density range (see Ch. 8, Sensitometry).

MANUFACTURING PROCESS

The manufacture of film is a complex physical and chemical process. A detailed understanding is not necessary, but a brief outline of the stages involved may help in the appreciation of topics such as photochemistry and sensitometry.

As stated previously, X-ray emulsions are mainly composed of silver bromide so we will now consider the manufacture of this material.

Silver bromide

Silver bromide is produced in the following reaction:

$$AgNO_3 + KBr \atop (excess) = AgBr \atop (insoluble) + KNO_3 \atop (soluble)$$

$$\frac{silver}{nitrate} + \frac{potassium}{bromide} = \frac{silver}{bromide} + \frac{potassium}{nitrate}$$

Emulsion manufacture can be divided into seven stages:

1. Emulsification
2. Physical ripening
3. Shredding
4. Washing
5. Chemical ripening
6. Doctoring
7. Coating.

These stages and the various imputs and extractions are illustrated in Figure 4.24. Many of the stages are under complex computer control to ensure accurate mixing and maintenance of temperatures, etc. All these processes must be carried out in complete darkness.

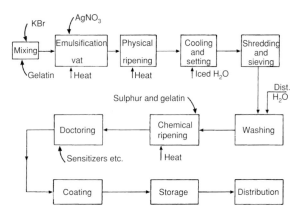

Fig. 4.24 Block diagram of the manufacturing process.

Emulsification

A mixture of gelatine and KBr is made in a large stainless steel vat to which is added the $AgNO_3$ solution, thus forming AgBr crystals. Continuous violent stirring ensures even mixing of the additives.

The temperature of the mixture and the rate of addition of the $AgNO_3$ solution determines the sizes of crystal produced, and varying the rate of addition has a strong effect on the contrast of the final emulsion.

Physical ripening

In this process the emulsion is stirred at a fixed temperature for a fixed length of time. This allows two processes to take place which allow an increase in the grain size of the mixture, causing an increase in sensitivity of the emulsion. Many factors influence this stage of manufacture including temperature, pH, concentration, time of ripening and the amount of agitation.

At the correct moment the emulsion is allowed to set by placing the vat in iced water.

Shredding

The solidified emulsion is then chopped into small 'noodles' and passed through a sieve into the fourth stage of the process.

Washing

This removes from the emulsion the soluble KNO_3 and the excess KBr, which would otherwise degrade its performance. Distilled running water is used, and the process usually takes 1–2 hours.

Chemical ripening

This increases the sensitivity of the emulsion by encouraging the build-up of 'sensitivity centres' within individual AgBr crystals. This increases the speed of the emulsion but does not alter the size and shape of the AgBr crystals.

The shredded, washed emulsion is re-melted and a proportion of gelatine that has been specially produced with high levels of sulphur impurities is mixed in. This mixture is then left at a temperature for a certain length of time, at the end of which chemical ripening is complete.

Doctoring

This is the stage at which all necessary additions are made to the emulsion to vary its characteristics:

1. *Sensitisers*
   These extend the spectral sensitivity of the emulsion from monochromatic to orthochromatic, panchromatic or infrared, as required.

2. *Hardener*
   Makes the emulsion resistant to abrasions, etc.

3. *Fungicide*
   Prevents the growth of bacteria and mould.

4. *Wetting agent*
   Reduces surface tension and allows easy penetration of chemicals.

5. *Plasticiser*
   Prevents the emulsion from becoming too brittle.

6. *Anti-foggant*
   Improves the keeping properties of the film.

7. *Anti-frothing agent*
   Prevents bubbles forming during coating.

Coating

The emulsion is now coated on either side of a base by a mechanical process, giving a thin, even layer. Modern base materials are nearly always polyester for standard X-ray film. This is pre-prepared by adding a thin coating of pure gelatine to act as an adhesive for the emulsion. After coating it is chilled, to set the emulsion, and left to dry. The final stage in the coating process is to add another layer of gelatine, called the supercoat, which protects the emulsion. The coating process is summarised in Figure 4.25.

The roll of film is now ready for slitting and packing into suitable containers. After packing, the fresh film is usually allowed to 'stand' for a few weeks to allow the silver bromide to stabilise. It is then ready for normal use.

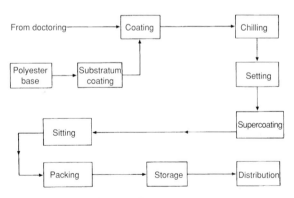

Fig. 4.25 Block diagram from coating to distribution.

REFERENCES

Penguin Dictionary of Physics 1979
Product information from Agfa Gevaert Ltd, 27 Great West Road, Brentford, Middlesex TW8 9AX
Product information from Fuji Photo Film (UK) Ltd, 125 Finchley Road, London NW3 6HY
Product information from Kodak Ltd, PO Box 66, Station Road, Hemel Hempstead, Herts HP1 1JU
Product information from Konica (UK) Ltd, Plane Tree Crescent, Feltham, Middlesex TW13 7HD

Chapter 5
Intensifying screens

INTRODUCTION

Radiography as we know it today would not be a viable proposition without the use of intensifying screens; exposures would be too long, giving excessive movement unsharpness, and the dose required to produce an acceptable image of most parts of the body would, to say the least, be too high.

Many improvements have taken place since the early days of radiography but until the early 1970s calcium tungstate intensifying screens were still the most widely used screens in radiography. Although other phosphors had been used, calcium tungstate remained the most suitable and its limitations prevented any major break-through in screen design.

In 1970, Wickersheim, Alves and Buchanan suggested the use of certain terbium-activated rare earth phosphors in intensifying screens and this proved to be the advance that screen technology had been waiting for, even though the early days were fraught with problems.

GENERAL CONSIDERATIONS

The remainder of this chapter is devoted almost entirely to consideration of calcium tungstate and rare earth phosphors, which are both now in common use. Certain areas which are common to both will be discussed before the specifics of each.

The need for screens

During exposure the X-ray beam is modified according to the structures through which it passes. The photons that have passed through the patient carry the information about that patient which then must be converted to a visual form.

Photographic emulsion exposed directly to these photons will record a suitable image. Unfortunately the sensitivity of film to direct X-ray exposure is very low and if used for all examinations would result in a prohibitively large X-ray dose and high movement unsharpness.

Intensifying screens convert the X-rays into visible light, which then exposes the film. This has the advantage of reducing the dose required for a particular examination, resulting in shorter exposure times and less movement unsharpness, but introduces other unsharpness problems due to screen structure (see Screen speed, p. 75 and Ch. 9, Image quality). As a generalisation, a film that is exposed using screens has an image that is produced 95% by light and 5% by X-rays, although this obviously depends on the particular technique used.

Screens are used as follows:

- Double screen technique, for example conventional radiography with duplitised X-ray film (see Ch. 4) in a cassette

- Single screen technique, for example mammography; usually in special cassette (e.g. vacuum cassette)

- Multiscreen techniques, for example tomographic multisection cassette.

What is a phosphor?

This is probably the first question that needs to be answered. In the Penguin *Dictionary of Science and Physics* (1979) it is defined as 'a substance that emits light at a temperature below the temperature at which it would exhibit incandescence'. This definition can be made more specific when considering phosphors for use in screens: a phosphor is usually a metallic crystalline solid, naturally occurring or artificially made, that exhibits the property of *fluorescence* when exposed to X-radiation and can be manufactured in useful form to produce high image quality.

Fluorescence has two closely allied terms associated with it, both of which are very easy to confuse. These terms are *luminescence* and *phosphorescence*. In order to fully understand the differences it is necessary to have some knowledge of the basic physics involved in these processes (see Luminescence: fluorescence and phosphorescence, p. 68).

How does a screen work?

Screens work by a three-stage process:

- Absorption
- Conversion
- Emission or re-emission.

Absorption

A great deal is known about the absorption processes. Any good physics textbook will discuss in some detail the photoelectric effect, Compton effect and pair production. In screens, the incident X-ray photons are absorbed in the phosphor material by either the photoelectric or the Compton effect. At energies used in diagnostic radiography the predominant effect is photoelectric. This occurs in the high atomic number elements of the phosphor and is further assisted by the fact that phosphors, being metallic crystalline solids, have a predominantly ionic structure which results in a low incidence of free electrons. In percentage terms the approximate number of photons absorbed by the photoelectric effect is 95%, to the Compton effect's 5%. In either case, secondary electrons are produced in relation to the exposure received (Fig. 5.1).

Conversion

In relation to the amount of knowledge about the absorption process, the conversion process is somewhat less clear. The energy available from the released electron is converted into light photons by either fluorescence or phosphorescence (see p. 68), both of which involve the movement of electrons between 'electron traps' and 'holes' within the 'forbidden gap' and 'conduction band' areas of the crystal (see Fig. 5.1).

Emission

Very little is known of the mechanisms of re-emission; of the three processes this is the least understood. Photons released by absorption and conversion leave the phosphor material and expose the film, producing the latent image and, after processing, a density that is proportional to their intensity. The wavelength of the emissions is controlled in manufacture so as to match as closely as possible the peak sensitivity of the film it is exposing (see Fig. 5.1).

CRYSTAL PHYSICS

The solid state physics contained within the next section is without mathematical formulae and is simplified.

Crystalline solids comprise a regular three-dimensional array of atoms or molecules. Figure 5.2. is an example of pure silver bromide, which has a cubic arrangement. Many different shapes are possible depending on the nature of the substance. The predominant bonding type is ionic bonding: this involves the transfer of electrons between atoms, resulting in positive and negative ions which then combine in a regular pattern to give a relatively stable configuration.

Energy levels

Within the stable configuration there are only certain allowable energy levels, or bands. These are determined by quantum mechanics. The three levels or allowed bands (Fig. 5.3) are:

- Valence band
- Forbidden band (or gap)
- Conduction band.

Valence band

In this band the electrons are so loosely bound to their parent nucleus that they are free for sharing by adjacent atoms or molecules.

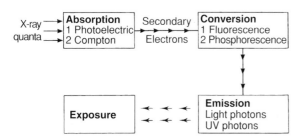

Fig. 5.1 Summary of screen function.

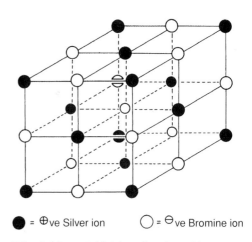

Fig. 5.2 Cubic crystal lattice: silver bromide.

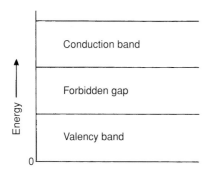

Fig. 5.3 Simplified energy level diagram.

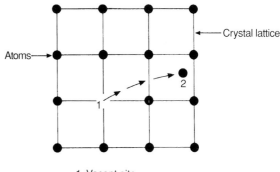

1. Vacant site
2. Interstitial ion/atom

Fig. 5.4 Frenkel defect.

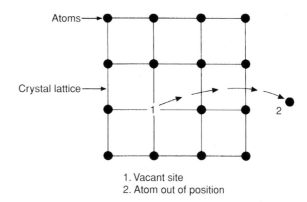

1. Vacant site
2. Atom out of position

Fig. 5.5 Schottky defect.

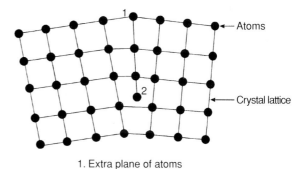

1. Extra plane of atoms
2. Dislocation extends into crystal

Fig. 5.6 Edge dislocation defect.

Forbidden band

Electrons within a system can only have a certain allowable range of energies. The forbidden band is the range of energies outside this allowable range. Electrons may 'pass through' this gap if they are energetic enough, but cannot exist in any form within this area.

Conduction band

Any electrons within this band are free to move providing they maintain a certain minimum energy. If they fall below this minimum, they return to the valence band or other vacant electron site.

If a potential difference is applied to a substance with electrons in its conduction band, an electric current can be made to flow.

Crystal defects

No system is perfect and crystals are no exception to this rule. Indeed, it is this departure from the perfect that enables the fluorescent and phosphorescent effects to take place. Departures from the regularity of the ionic structure are called *defects* and are of two main types:

1. Point defects
   —Frenkel defect (Fig. 5.4)
   —Schottky defect (Fig. 5.5)

2. Line defects
   —Edge dislocations (Fig. 5.6)
   —Screw dislocation.

These defects create areas of low energy within the crystal, called 'electron traps' and 'holes'.

Even supposedly perfect crystals contain some defects. The number of defects rises exponentially with temperature, typical values for point defects being 1 in 10^5 at 700°C for metals (i.e. 1 site in 100 000 is vacant). Defects can be produced by heating followed by rapid cooling, by pressure and by ionising radiations.

Traps

Traps are areas of low energy within the crystal that have the ability to catch and hold an electron for a period of time until it acquires the energy to escape.

The escape energy may be small (as in silver bromide) or very high (as in lithium fluoride). Traps are usually caused by two adjacent atoms attempting to share the charge of another atom, and are mainly the result of line-type defects.

Holes

A hole is the absence of an electron in the valence band; it is regarded as a mobile vacancy and has a positive electronic charge equal to that of a proton. Although it is a space left by an electron, it is regarded as a positive charge as the 'hole' has the ability to attract an electron.

Luminescence: fluorescence and phosphorescence (Figs 5.7, 5.8)

As previously indicated, these topics are central to the way a screen functions. They are often con-fused, perhaps owing to their obvious similarity in pronunciation. It is as well to note that the actual mechanisms involved in the production of these three phenomena are still not clearly understood and, therefore, any discussion is limited to theory only.

Luminescence

This can be radiographically defined as the ability of a substance to absorb short wavelength radiation and emit longer wavelength radiation, normally within the visible or near-visible spectrum. More generally it is the emission of electromagnetic radiation from a substance as the result of any non-thermal process.

Luminescence comprises two effects:

• Fluorescence
• Phosphorescence (or after-glow).

Fluorescence

A material is said to fluoresce when light emission starts when the exciting radiation starts, and light emission stops when the exciting radiation stops. This, however, is somewhat simplified, as

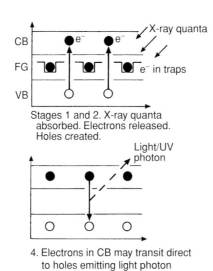

Stages 1 and 2. X-ray quanta absorbed. Electrons released. Holes created.

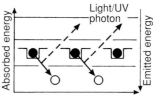

3. Electrons in traps transit to holes. Light photons emitted.

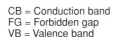

4. Electrons in CB may transit direct to holes emitting light photon

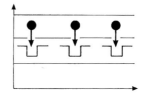

5. Vacancies in traps filled by electrons from CB.

CB = Conduction band
FG = Forbidden gap
VB = Valence band

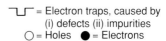

= Electron traps, caused by (i) defects (ii) impurities
○ = Holes ● = Electrons

Fig. 5.7 Fluorescence: diagrammatic representation.

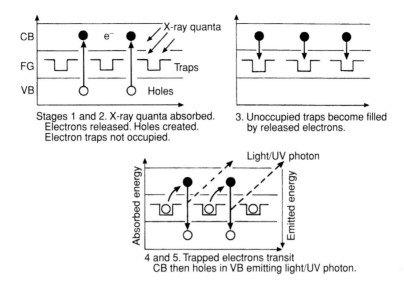

Fig. 5.8 Phosphorescence: diagrammatic representation.

even in the quickest responding phosphor there is some time lag before peak emission is reached and some light emission after the exposure has stopped. If this lag and continued emission is less than 10^{-8} seconds then the phosphor is said to fluoresce. The value of 10^{-8} seconds is used as this approximately corresponds to the time taken for an electron transition between energy levels to produce a light photon (see Fig. 5.9).

The physical process of fluorescence can be described by considering Figure 5.7. Incoming X-ray energy is absorbed, producing secondary electrons. If these electrons have sufficient energy they transit the forbidden band and become free in the conduction band. This leaves 'holes' in the valence band. These 'holes' are immediately filled by electrons, either directly from the conduction band or from the electron traps within the forbidden band. The transition results in yet another energy change that produces a light photon. To complete the process, any vacant trap in the forbidden band is now able to capture free electrons from the conduction band.

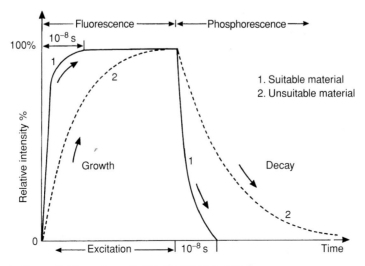

Fig. 5.9 Diagram illustrating suitable and unsuitable phosphor material.

This does not produce a light photon, as the energy change is too small.

Phosphorescence or after-glow

After-glow is the continuation of light emission even though the exciting radiation has stopped. Again, the threshold value is 10^{-8} seconds, and if a phosphor takes longer than this value to reach peak emission or if it continues to emit light after this period it is considered to phosphoresce (see Fig. 5.9).

The physical process can be described by considering Figure 5.8. As with fluorescence, the incoming X-ray is absorbed producing secondary electrons that, providing they possess sufficient energy, may become free in the conduction band. This creates 'holes' in the valence band. The free electrons then fall into traps where they are held for a period of time (determined by crystal type and inherent impurities). If the trapped electron acquires enough energy it will escape from the trap and return to the holes in the valence band either directly or via the conduction band. In either case the energy change produces a light photon.

It is the holding of the electron in a trap for a 'period of time' that is the cause of the after-glow, as even when the exciting radiation stops there will still be some electrons waiting to transit between bands.

The length of delay in the emission is determined by the time taken for the electron to escape from its trap and return to a 'hole' in the valence band. It is logical therefore that this also determines how long light is emitted after excitation ceases.

Phosphorescence in screens is an undesirable effect, as it causes multi-imaging and occasionally film fogging. Unfortunately, it is not possible to differentiate completely between the two effects, and all screens have some after-glow (even though this may be so slight as to be insignificant from a practical point of view).

After-glow can sometimes be useful: for example, in an oscilloscope the path of a 'single dot' trace can still be seen even though the dot has moved on; it is the basis of so-called luminous dials on clocks and watches, and finally it is useful in dose meters where re-emission of the light photons does not occur until the material has been heated to a certain temperature (thermoluminescent dosimetry).

Some terminology

Figure 5.9 illustrates some of the common terminology associated with phosphor technology and also shows the fluorescent and phosphorescent processes in terms of a material that may be suitable for screen manufacture and one that is not suitable. Both have a growth and decay period, and the duration of that period defines one criterion for a phosphor's suitability in screen manufacture. Other factors would be spectral emission, resolution, speed, manufacturing suitability, etc.

Dopants

These are impurities that are introduced into the phosphor crystal structure in order to control its characteristics. Dopants are normally one of two kinds:

- Activators
- Killers.

Activators

Activators are impurities that stimulate the phosphor to emit light. Careful choice of the amount and type of activator enables the spectral emission of the phosphor to be controlled so it can be tailored to match the peak sensitivity of the film it is intended to expose. Only one phosphor in use in radiography does not require an activator: that is calcium tungstate, which is considered to be 'self-activating'. All of the others require the presence of a dopant in order to emit light; for example, lanthanum oxybromide (LaOBr) does not fluoresce unless it has a small percentage of activator present (usually terbium (Tb)). Conventionally the activator is written after the main phosphor formula and following a full stop, e.g. terbium-activated lanthanum oxybromide is written LaOBr.Tb.

Killers

This form of dopant is not used a great deal in screen technology. It is introduced to the phosphor structure to control the areas of the crystal responsible for phosphorescence and is therefore used to control after-glow.

Some phosphors may contain both activators and killers in order to produce a viable material.

SUMMARY

Introduction and basic physics

- Screens are used principally to reduce the amount of X-ray exposure the patient receives. Screens convert incoming X-ray photons into light.

- The image produced on the film is produced 95% by light and 5% by X-rays (approximately).

- The screen phosphor must possess the property of fluorescence.

- Screens function by absorption, conversion and emission:

   Absorption is mainly due to the photoelectric effect.
   Conversion is either by fluorescence or phosphorescence.
   These involve the movement of electrons between traps and 'holes'.
   Emission is controlled to match the peak sensitivity of the film the screen is going to expose.

- Crystal physics, including energy levels, valence band, forbidden band, conduction band, crystal defects, traps, holes, etc., can be found in the text.

- Luminescence is the ability of a substance to absorb short wavelength radiation and emit longer wavelength radiation in the visible or near-visible spectrum. Luminescence comprises two effects, fluorescence and phosphorescence (after-glow):

   Fluorescence is when the light emission ceases when the exciting radiation ceases.
   Phosphorescence is when light continues to be emitted after the exciting radiation ceases. After-glow can cause unsharpness of the image.

- Dopants can be divided into activators and killers:

   Activators are impurities that are added to a phosphor to stimulate it to emit light.
   Killers are added to try to control after-glow.

CONSTRUCTION OF SCREENS

An intensifying screen is constructed of various layers, as shown in Figure 5.10.

Base

This acts as a support for all the other layers and is made of polyester. In many cases it is the same material as that used for film base but without the coloured tint. Base thickness varies but is approximately 250 microns (μ) for screens used in cassettes, and may be as thin as 175 μ for screens used in automatic film changers. The reflective or absorptive layer is usually incorporated in the upper part of the base, although it is separated in Figure 5.10 because of its functional significance.

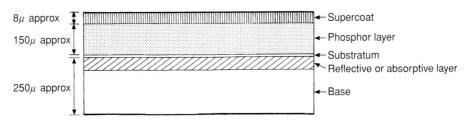

Fig. 5.10 Typical cross-sectional structure of a universal intensifying screen. All dimensions approximate.

Most base materials have been developed after many years of expensive research, and are therefore heavily protected by patents held by their manufacturers.

Reflective or absorptive layer

This layer does exactly as its name suggests. As phosphor crystals emit light in all directions, a significant proportion of that light is going away from the film. The *reflective layer* redirects it towards the film, therefore ensuring that it contributes to exposure.

Advantages

- Increasing the speed of the film/screen combination
- A corresponding reduction in patient dose.

Disadvantage

- Increasing the amount of unsharpness produced (see Speed, p. 75, and Resolution, p. 81).

In many screens the reflective layer is a thin coating (30 μ) of titanium dioxide (TiO_2) or similar compound.

If the layer is *absorptive*, light travelling away from the film is absorbed by a dye and does not contribute to the formation of the image.

Advantage

- Improves the sharpness of the image.

Disadvantage

- Slows down the speed of the system.

The *dyes* used in this layer are the subject of complicated patents, each manufacturer using its own particular development even though the chemical formulae may be very similar.

Substratum

This is effectively a layer of 'glue' that is used to attach the phosphor layer to the base. It is made as thin as coating technology will allow with regard to providing adequate adhesion between the two layers.

Phosphor layer

This is a suspension of the phosphor crystals within a suitable binder. It is approximately 150 μ thick in universal screens.

Binder technology is complex. A binder must be:

- Flexible
- Inert to the phosphor crystals and the light they emit
- Provide even, known dispersion of the phosphor in the binder
- Able to be coated, with the phosphor, onto the base at the required thickness.

Most manufacturers use acetate acrylate as the binding agent, as this has all the necessary characteristics.

Phosphor characteristics

- Even *dispersion* of the phosphor is vital, as areas of high concentration would lead to uneven light emission from the screen and consequent uneven exposure of the film.

- Each phosphor crystal is completely surrounded by the binder and the amount of phosphor per unit volume is known; this amount is called the *coating weight*, and is determined during manufacture.

The relevance of this is that a screen with a high coating weight (i.e. a high amount of phosphor per unit volume) can be made thinner, and therefore produce a sharper image, than a screen with a lower coating weight in the same speed class (see Speed, p. 75, and Resolution, p. 81).

Some modern screens have a high pigment to binder ratio referred to as 'light piping'. This enables more light to be emitted by the phosphor resulting in a sharper image being produced.

- The *specific gravity* of the phosphor. In theory, the higher the specific gravity, the thinner the phosphor layer can be for any given speed class, but in practice the phosphor/binder relationship is found to be more significant in determining phosphor thickness. In universal screens, the ratio is approximately 9 parts phosphor to 1 part binder. Screen speed is also determined in the phosphor layer, the general rule being that, within limits, the thicker the phosphor the more light it will produce, and therefore the more exposure the film will receive for the same dose.

However, the addition of coloured dyes to the binder means speed and resolution can be controlled without altering the phosphor thickness (see Speed, p. 75, and Resolution, p. 81).

Supercoat

This is the top protective layer of the screen. It is usually a thin coating (about 8 µ) of cellulose acetobiturate which:

- Protects the phosphor layer from mechanical damage
- Provides a surface that is easy to clean
- Is a poor generator of static electricity.

It has been estimated that a static charge of up to 4 kV can be generated by sliding a film quickly over that surface of a screen as it is removed from the cassette. Static marks will therefore appear on the film causing artefacts. Modern developments have introduced electron beam cured topcoats which enable a thinner, more protective supercoat giving the screens a longer life and increasing image sharpness:

- The surface of the supercoat can be made with varying degrees of 'roughness'. For example, a *smooth surface* screen (i.e. one with a low friction coefficient) would be of little use in an automatic film changer as the film would slide through the screens before they have a chance to close and 'trap' the film.

- A totally smooth surface tends to trap air between the film and screen in the cassette, causing poor film/screen contact.

- Too rough a surface can seriously degrade image quality by increasing screen unsharpness factors.

The degree of screen 'roughness' (or friction coefficient) is therefore carefully controlled to suit the situation the screen will be used in. This is particularly important with the increased use of automated film handling systems such as 'film centres' and 'daylight systems'.

INTENSIFYING FACTOR (IF)

This is defined as the ratio of the exposure required to produce net density (ND) 1.0 without screens using a particular film, compared to the exposure required to produce net density 1.0 using screens with the same film, i.e:

$$\text{IF} = \frac{\text{Exposure required to produce ND 1.0: No screens}}{\text{Exposure required to produce ND 1.0: Screens}}$$

Conventionally, net density 1.0 is used as this is a convenient point approximately halfway up the characteristic curve (see Sensitometry, p. 155); however, any density is a perfectly acceptable alternative providing that this is stated in the calculation, does not exceed the maximum useful density and is above the minimum useful density.

Effectively the IF of a screen tells you by how much you can reduce the exposure required to produce a particular film if you put that same film in screens.

For example, if a radiograph has been taken using a direct exposure technique, and the exposure required to produce an acceptable image was 50 kV, 25 mAs at 100 cm focus-film distance (ffd) – what exposure factors would be required to achieve the same image if a screen film combination with an IF5 was used?

Using the above formula:

$$5 = \frac{25}{\text{Exposure required using screen}}$$

$$= 5\,\text{mAs}$$

Therefore the new exposure would be 5 mAs.

This technique also allows changes in exposure between two screens of known IF to be calculated, again providing the same film is used. For example:

$$\text{Change to exposure factors} = \frac{\text{Original IF}}{\text{New IF}}$$

If a screen film combination with an IF of 10 was introduced into a department, replacing intensifying screens with a factor of 5, how would the exposure factors be changed to produce the equivalent image?

Using the above formula:

$$\text{Change to exposure factors} = \frac{5}{10}$$

$$= 0.5$$

Therefore the mAs would be reduced by a factor of 0.5.

To be completely accurate, IF should be quoted at a particular kV value or range of values. This is because the absorption of X-ray photons in the screen depends principally on the value, in photon energy, kiloelectron volts (keV), of the K absorption edge of the heavy element present in the phosphor. If the energy of the X-ray photon is at this value (or values for other significant absorption edges), then the degree of photoelectric absorption will be high and, in general, the amount of light emitted will also be increased compared to the amount released by photons with a marginally higher or lower energy (in most cases the higher the absorption, the higher the light output, the faster the screens and the higher the IF; see Screen speed, p. 75).

This leads to the conclusion that all screens are kV dependent. As an example, Figure 5.11 shows

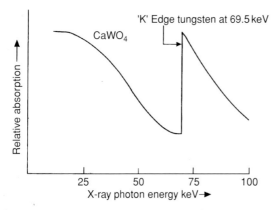

Fig. 5.11 Illustration of the photoelectric absorption properties of calcium tungstate and how it varies with X-ray photon energy.

the K absorption edge for calcium tungstate. Between 15 and 69.5 keV there is a fall in the relative photoelectric absorption. At 69.5 keV there is a massive jump in absorption which again starts to tail off as the photon energy increases towards 100 keV.

When using calcium tungstate screens in the 60–90 kV range:

An increase in exposure of 10 kV allows an approximate reduction in mAs of one-half, and will still produce a film of similar density

(i.e. 50 mAs, 70 kV is equal to 25 mAs, 80 kV in terms of film blackening).

In order to emphasise the importance of the intensification properties of screens, consider one X-ray photon falling on a direct exposure film. If this is absorbed by the film it will produce one development centre when the film is processed (see Ch. 6, Photochemistry). If the same photon is absorbed by a high speed calcium tungstate screen it will produce approximately 800 light photons; about half of these are absorbed in the screen before they reach the film, leaving 400 photons to expose the film.

If it takes, say, 10 light photons to produce one development centre, then the number of development centres produced is approximately equal to 40. This does not mean exposure reductions of × 40 are required when going from no-screen to screen techniques, but illustrates that the amplifying power of screens is considerable (see Screen speed, p. 75).

SUMMARY

Construction and intensification factor

A cross-sectional diagram of the construction of a *screen* is shown in Figure 5.10. It consists of:

- *Base*
  Made from polyester, approximately 250 μ thick. Similar to film base.

- *Reflective absorptive layer*
  Either absorbs or reflects light emitted by the screen phosphor. This significantly affects

screen speed and unsharpness. If reflective, it is a layer of titanium dioxide or similar compound.

- *Phosphor layer*
  This is a suspension of phosphor crystals in a suitable binder. Binder technology is extremely complex. Most manufacturers use acetate acrylate as the binding agent.

- *Supercoat*
  Top protective layer of the screen, it is a very thin coating of cellulose acetobiturate or similar material. The supercoat may be completely smooth or deliberately roughened, depending on the use to which the screen will be put.

Intensification factor is defined as the ratio of the exposure required to produce net density 1.0 without screens using a particular film, compared to the exposure required to produce the same density using screens with the same film: i.e. by how much you can reduce the exposure when moving from a direct exposure to a screen technique.

SCREEN SPEED AND DETAIL

Screen speed and detail are inexorably linked. The general relationship is a reciprocal one; that is, as the speed of a film/screen combination increases, the amount of detail decreases (i.e. there is an increase in unsharpness: see Ch. 9, Image quality).

The main factors affecting speed are listed below. Each factor is then discussed in turn and its effect on detail is considered either within the section or (if more appropriate) at the end.

- Phosphor type – efficiency
- Thickness of phosphor layer/coating weight
- Presence of absorptive/reflective layer
- Presence of dye in phosphor binder or supercoat
- Exposure technique
- Phosphor grain size.

Phosphor type

Different phosphors used in screens can affect their speed. For example, it is generally accepted that rare earth screens are 'faster' than calcium tungstate ($CaWO_4$) screens; however, this is an oversimplification. It is possible to make rare earth screens and calcium tungstate screens of the same speed class (see Speed class, p. 79) but one will produce quite different results in terms of resolution compared to the other.

For example, if the same amounts, in terms of volume, of calcium tungstate and a rare earth phosphor were subject to exactly the same X-ray exposure, and the light given off exposed a film that was of the correct spectral sensitivity to record the emission, it would be found, in general, that the film exposed to the rare earth phosphor would have a higher density than the film exposed to calcium tungstate.

The amount of light output from screens is normally examined by considering their efficiency. It has already been stated that screens work by the three stage process of absorption, conversion and emission. Total efficiency is the product of the efficiency of each of the processes, so that:

$$N_t = N_a \times N_c \times N_e$$

where:

N_t = Total efficiency
N_a = Absorption efficiency
N_c = Conversion efficiency
N_e = Emission efficiency.

Absorption efficiency is also known as quantum detection efficiency (QDE). Both terms are equally valid when considering the total efficiency of a screen system.

The value of the emission efficiency may be omitted, as this considerably simplifies quantitative evaluation due to the fact that this value is difficult to calculate!

Total efficiency can be increased by increasing any one of the three variables or any combination of them.

In general, the mother crystal determines the absorption, while the dopant determines the conversion; therefore, changing from a low absorption self-doped crystal (such as $CaWO_4$) to a high absorption deliberately doped crystal (such as LaOBr.Tb) results in increased efficiency, increased light output and apparently higher speed. The type of re-emission from the crystal is

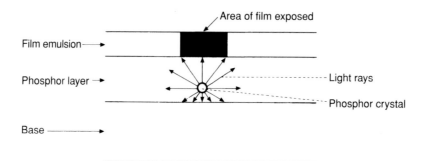

Fig. 5.12 Unsharpness due to screens: area of film exposed greater than that of the phosphor crystal.

thought to be determined by its shape – but precisely how, in most cases, is not clear.

Phosphor thickness

This is the factor that contributes most to screen unsharpness. The general rule is that:

For the same phosphor type, the thicker the phosphor layer, the faster the screen but the greater the unsharpness it produces.

Consider Figure 5.12. Suppose an incoming X-ray photon causes a phosphor crystal that is far away from the film to emit light. This light is given off in all directions but only some of it reaches the film. As can be seen from the figure, the area of film exposed is larger than the phosphor crystal. This amount of spread of the light due to the distance it has travelled can be qualitatively expressed by the value 'u' in Figure 5.13. If the thickness of the phosphor is increased, the value of 'u' also increases (Fig. 5.14(i)) and the unsharpness produced increases.

However, if the phosphor is thicker, more of the incoming X-ray photons will be absorbed, the total efficiency will increase and more light photons will be given off. Consequently, to produce a similar film density a reduction in exposure will be required, i.e. the screen has increased in speed. The converse is also true, in that, for the same phosphor type:

The thinner the layer, the slower the screen but the less the unsharpness.

It is not possible to go on increasing screen speed by this method indefinitely. Apart from the problems of unsharpness, an optimum value of screen thickness to coating weight of crystal is reached which produces the highest light output. Exceeding this optimum eventually results in the screen absorbing its own light output with the effect that no increase in speed results from using a thicker phosphor layer.

Other relevant factors to be considered are the presence or absence of an absorptive dye in the phosphor binder or reflective layer. For example, if speed control is being exercised by dye tinting, then two screens which have the same thickness may have different speed and unsharpness factors, due to the presence of the dye.

Coating weight

This is the amount of phosphor present per unit volume. The basic principle is quite simple in that the more phosphor crystals there are in a given volume, the more light will be emitted due to the higher chance of X-ray absorption in that volume. Therefore:

The higher the coating weight, the faster the screen.

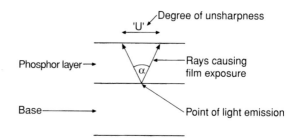

Fig. 5.13 Screen unsharpness: quantitative approach.

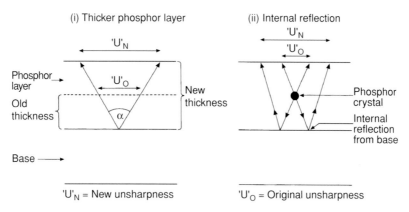

'U'$_N$ = New unsharpness   'U'$_O$ = Original unsharpness

Fig. 5.14 Screen unsharpness: (i) thicker phosphor layer; (ii) internal reflection.

The amount of phosphor present depends on the specific gravity of the phosphor and the phosphor/binder ratio. In theory the higher the specific gravity, the higher the coating weight possible, but in practice the phosphor/binder ratio is more significant in determining speed and unsharpness.

Reflective/absorptive layer

As detailed earlier, these layers are coated on top of the base. If the layer is *reflective*, any light going away from the film is redirected towards the film and contributes to its exposure:

The effective speed of the screen is increased but so is unsharpness.

This is due to the internal reflection increasing the 'u' value as shown in Figure 5.14(ii).

The action of the *absorptive layer* is exactly the opposite of that of the reflective layer. It is normally a coloured dye that absorbs light going away from the film:

This reduces the speed of the screen (because of the reduction in light reaching the film) and also reduces the degree of unsharpness.

The use of an absorption layer as described here is a relatively rare way of controlling screen speed.

It is quite possible for there to be neither of these layers present. When this is the case, some internal reflections still occur due to the boundary between the base and the phosphor layer, and this still contributes to speed and unsharpness.

Dye tint in binder

This is probably the most common way to control screen speed and unsharpness. Its principle is based on the inclusion of a coloured dye within the binder of the phosphor layer and the effect that this has on the amount of light reaching the film. It is described quantitively by the *Beer–Lambert law* which states: 'The proportion of light absorbed by a medium varies exponentially with the product of the path length of the light in the medium, the molar concentration and the molecular extinction coefficient.' In other words:

The greater the distance a ray of light travels in a coloured medium, the more it is absorbed.

The effect this has on screen speed and resolution is illustrated in Figure 5.15. It shows a phosphor crystal producing a degree of unsharpness ('u') due to lateral diffusion of the light represented by angle α. The distance the light has travelled is represented by 'x'. If a coloured dye is added to the binder, the value of 'u' decreases because the amount of light absorbed by the dye in transiting the path length ('x') is such that only a very small fraction (or none at all) reaches and exposes the film. In order for sufficient light to reach the film to produce an appreciable image, the path length ('x') must decrease. This can only

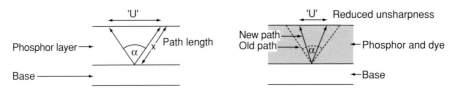

Fig. 5.15 Screen unsharpness: reduction due to dye tinting phosphor layer.

occur if angle α gets smaller and this in turn results in a reduction in the unsharpness ('u').

The result of this on speed is that, as the dye has a light-absorbing effect, it reduces the exposure reaching the film. This must be compensated for by increase in exposure in order to obtain a similar film density, providing the same film is used.

A similar effect can be obtained by placing the dye in the supercoat; however, this is somewhat limited in terms of its effectiveness and is rarely used.

Exposure technique

The rare earth phosphors are 'kV dependent'. In practice this means that in order to make the best use of their total efficiency it is necessary to use them within a certain kV range.

Consider Figure 5.16. This shows how relative speed varies against kVp set for five different systems:

1. A BaFCl.Eu system of speed class 350–400 (approximately)

2. A Gd_2O_2S.Tb system of speed class 150–400 (approximately)

3. A Gd_2O_2S.Tb system of speed class 130–240 (approximately)

4. A LaOBr.Tb system of speed class 150–200 (approximately)

5. A $CaWO_4$ system (which is represented as a straight line for ease of comparison) of speed class 100.

For example, *system 3* has its maximum speed at approximately 90 kV (speed class 240) with quite a marked fall off at kVs higher and lower than this. If this system was used in a situation requiring a set kV of, say, 70 kV, then its speed class will have fallen to 200.

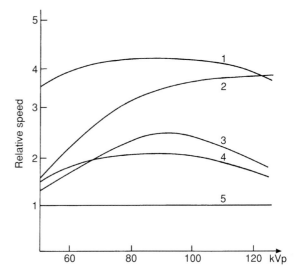

Fig. 5.16 System speed variation with kV.

System 4, however, has quite a flat top to its curve, illustrating that this system maintains its speed class of 200 quite well between 70 and 95 kV but either side of this limit it falls away until, for example, at 55 kV its speed is not much better than $CaWO_4$.

In practice, it is important to know how the speed of a screen varies with the kV selected, as this could significantly influence the choice of what film/screen system should be used for a particular examination.

One final point to be considered is that Figure 5.16 implies that $CaWO_4$ screens are not kV dependent. This is not the case, but their dependency on variation in kV is not as marked as that of their competitors and is often represented as a straight line for comparative purposes.

Phosphor grain size

Phosphor grain size is of theoretical concern only, the principle being that, within certain limits, the larger the phosphor grain, the greater its absorption and therefore the more light it will emit. If a phosphor layer was made up of large grains it would be faster but produce more unsharpness than if the screen were made up of smaller grains, all other factors staying equal. In practice phosphor grains in screens have a range of sizes; these are usually 4–8 µ in commercially available systems.

The fact that no matter what speed class a particular screen falls into it will have a phosphor grain size of 4–8 µ is quite reasonable, as the manufacture of even this range of accuracy of size is quite a complex process. Considering this with the previously listed factors affecting speed, it is easy to see that the use of phosphor grain size in speed control in practical systems is of little concern, providing they are small enough to provide adequate sharpness.

General interrelation of speed factors

The interrelationships of the factors affecting speed and detail are numerous, complex and the subject of much discussion. Complete consideration of all of these factors is not within the scope of this chapter, but to illustrate the complexities involved consider the following question:

Two different film/screen combinations have the same speed class of 200. The first is a calcium tungstate system with conventional RP film, the second is a rare earth lanthanum oxybromide system with the same film. Which would you expect to produce the better image detail?

Both systems are the same speed class so they require the same exposure to produce similar image densities. The LaOBr.Tb has greater total efficiency than the $CaWO_4$ system, so in order to

get the same amount of exposure to the film, two options are open:

1. The phosphor layer can be made thinner, or

2. The phosphor layer can remain the same thickness but have a dye introduced so as to reduce the speed to that of the $CaWO_4$ system.

In either case, the amount of unsharpness produced by the rare earth system is less, so it appears to be the best choice. However, other questions also need to be asked, for example:

*   How thick is the supercoat?

*   What about quantum mottle?

*   What about the effect of other unsharpness factors such as focal spot size, focus-film distance, etc.?

As can be seen, the answer to a relatively simple question such as which combination produces the best detail is a far from simple.

Speed classification

One of the major problems concerning film/screen combinations has been the difficulty in comparing different manufacturer's systems in terms of their speed. This has been accentuated with the introduction of so-called half-speed film, orthochromatic and monochromatic rare earth systems and high speed barium fluorochloride phosphors.

The use of *speed class* considerably simplifies this problem and allows easy comparison of systems in terms of speed (but not necessarily of detail rendition). It is based on an arbitrary scale, with the value 100 being the benchmark to which all other systems are compared.

Table 5.1 illustrates the basis of the system. As can be seen, the speed classes range from 50 up to 800.

Table 5.1 Speed classification: system basics					
Speed class	50	100	200	400	800
Required mAs* changes to produce similar densities (fixed kV + ffd)	200 mAs	100 mAs	50 mAs	25 mAs	12.5 mAs
Exposure alteration compared to class 100	×2	1	$\frac{1}{2}$	$\frac{1}{4}$	$\frac{1}{8}$

* All mAs values are approximate.

Values intermediate to those shown are often found (e.g. speed class 350), as also are values higher and lower (e.g. 1200 and 25), but conventionally most systems fall into the range illustrated. The advantage of using speed class now comes into its own, as apart from showing relative system speed it also shows the variation in exposure required when changing from one system to another.

For example: you are at present using a speed class 100 system and the exposure required to produce a particular image is 70 kV 100 mAs 90 cm ffd. In order to produce a *similar* image, the following would be required:

- If you use a speed class 200 system, then the exposure would be 70 kV 50 mAs 90 cm ffd
- If it was a 400 system the mAs would be 25 mAs, or
- If class 50, 200 mAs.

Therefore, as the speed class goes up, the amount of exposure required to produce an image goes down compared to lower speed class values.

A note of caution is perhaps required here:

1. As the relationships are only approximate it is not always possible to produce an exactly similar image in terms of the densities produced. This is mainly due to the kV dependency of the phosphors and other factors that are not relevant at this time. However, the approximations hold true for many practical purposes.

2. As previously stated, a lower speed class does not necessarily mean improved image quality, as phosphor type and screen structure are not considered. For example, a rare earth system speed class 200 may produce equal or better detail than a $CaWO_4$ speed class 100 due to factors previously discussed.

A *general* rule that seems to hold true is that rare earth systems, compared to other systems in the same speed class, produce better detail radiographs.

A final note is that not all manufacturers use the designators 100, 200, etc.: some use 1, 2, 4, 8, and so on, but the interrelationship is the same (i.e. 4–8 is halving the exposure).

SUMMARY

Screen speed and detail

- In general as screen speed increases there is decrease in image detail, providing the same phosphor is being used. It must be remembered that this is not always the case.

- The main factors affecting speed and detail are:
  Phosphor type
  Thickness of the phosphor layer and *coating weight*
  Presence of *absorptive or reflective layer*
  Dye tinting of the binder or supercoat
  Exposure technique.

- *Phosphor type*
  The higher the total efficiency of the phosphor the more light output the phosphor will produce, providing similar amounts of phosphor are being considered. The rare earth phosphors gain an increase in overall efficiency by having a high absorption efficiency compared to that of calcium tungstate (see Table 5.3). The more efficient the phosphor, the thinner it can be coated to produce the same speed class and, as a result, the higher the image sharpness it will give.

- *Phosphor thickness*
  In general, the thicker the phosphor, the faster the screen and the greater the unsharpness it will produce (see Figs 5.13, 5.14). However, dye tinting may alter this simple relationship.

- *Coating weight*
  This is the amount of phosphor per unit volume. It depends on the phosphor's specific gravity and on the phosphor/binder ratio.

- *Reflective/absorptive layer*
  The reflective layer increases screen speed but also increases unsharpness (as a result of internal reflection; see Fig. 5.14(ii)). The absorptive layer decreases screen speed but also decreases unsharpness. These layers may or may not be present.

- *Dye tinting*
  This is the most common way to control screen speed and unsharpness. The addition of a

coloured dye to the binder reduces screen speed and increases the sharpness by reducing the 'u' value, as shown in Figure 5.15. Occasionally the supercoat may be tinted to produce a similar effect, but this is done only rarely.

- *Exposure technique*
  This has no effect on screen unsharpness but can have effects on screen speed. Rare earth phosphors are 'kV dependent' and have their highest speed within a certain range of kilovoltages. Careful selection of exposure factors enables the highest speed to be obtained (see Fig. 5.16).

- *Speed classification*
  This is a method of comparing film/screen combinations in terms of their relative speed. It allows different manufacturers' systems to be classified in such a way as to make changing from one to another, in terms of what exposures to use, a simple process.

CROSSOVER EFFECT

This effect occurs due to the use of duplitised film emulsions and is a feature of single or multi-screen techniques. It produces a decrease in image quality caused by the light, which is not completely absorbed in the first emulsion layer, passing through the base and exposing the second emulsion layer (Fig. 5.17). This significantly contributes to unsharpness, as can be seen qualitatively in the figure.

The widening light beam is the result of light diffusion within the grains as it passes from one side to the other, causing a 'wider', less sharp image in the emulsion layer furthest away from the initial light emission.

The degree of crossover is usually expressed as a percentage, and varies from 15–25% in ultraviolet/blue systems to 60% in orthochromatic systems. More formally, crossover can be defined as:

The amount of light transmitted to the opposite side of the base expressed as a percentage. (Fig. 5.18)

Image degradation caused by 60% crossover is so great that it may necessitate the inclusion of an

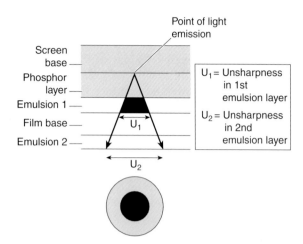

Fig. 5.17 Crossover effect: showing unsharpness reduced in two emulsion layers.

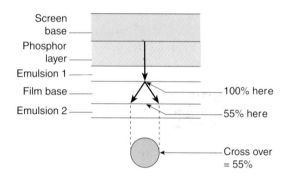

Fig. 5.18 Crossover effect: calculation of percentage crossover.

anti-halation layer, or anti-halation 'in coating', as part of the film structure in order to reduce it to an acceptable level. In turn, this may mean that only a particular film should be used with a particular screen in order to obtain the best results. This makes the film screen combination a so-called 'closed system'.

RESOLUTION

Resolution is measured in *line pairs per millimetre* (lp mm^{-1}) but is quite often seen as line pairs per centimetre or even line pairs per inch.

A line pair is a line of a particular width followed by a space of the same width; so, for example, if the quoted resolution for a particular system is 4 lp mm^{-1}, this means that there are four lines and spaces contained within 1 mm, therefore each line is 0.125 mm wide and each space is 0.125 mm wide. Therefore:

> **Resolution indicates the size of the smallest object that the system will record and, therefore, the smallest distance that must exist between two objects before they are seen as two separate objects.**

Typical values for resolution are 6–8 lp mm^{-1} for speed class 100, and 4–6 lp mm^{-1} for speed class 200 and 400. Unfortunately resolution gives:

- No indication of a system's performance in recording the detail of objects larger than the limiting resolution
- No indication how the system copes with high or low contrast details.

Resolution may be quoted either for the system resolution (i.e. the X-ray equipment plus film/screen combination plus processing, etc.) or it may be a theoretically calculated value.

It is also important to distinguish between resolution (which is objective) and definition (which is subjective). For more detail see Chapter 9, Image quality.

MOTTLE

This is the 'granular' appearance in areas of seemingly even density in the radiographic image. Contributors to this can be conveniently divided into three sections:

- Film grain
- Quantum mottle
- Structure mottle.

Film grain

> **Film grain is due to the coarse structure of the silver crystals forming the overall density in the emulsion.**

Even though the silver halide crystals are small (10^{-6} m), development tends to make them aggregate together (clumping) and form a small but visible unevenness in density. Many factors can affect this, ranging from film speed to processing conditions. True film grain in modern emulsions is so small as to be almost imperceptible, but it can be seen on magnification.

A fuller description of grain is to be found in Chapter 9, Image quality.

Quantum mottle

Sometimes called 'noise':

> **Quantum mottle is due to the random distribution of image-forming X-ray quanta producing non-uniform light emission from the screens.**

This light subsequently exposes the film, producing a developable silver halide grain or grains. In general the faster the film/screen combination is, the higher the quantum mottle will be because the lower the dose required to produce a given density, the fewer X-ray quanta there will be and the higher the chance that these will be recorded on the film as a separate 'density spot'.

However, this does not take into account the fact that one film may have high quantum mottle compared to another film but it may be less well 'imaged', i.e. unsharp, and consequently less visible.

True quantum mottle is a significant degree coarser than true film grain.

A fuller description of quantum mottle is to be found in Chapter 9, Image quality.

Structure mottle

This is a feature of the screen manufacturing process:

> **Structure mottle is caused by the fact that it is not possible to evenly disperse the phosphor crystals throughout the binder medium.**

No matter how efficient the mixing and coating process, areas of high phosphor crystal density occur. When exposed, these areas produce a higher light output than the surrounding areas and consequently a higher film density. This contributes to the overall mottled appearance.

In practice, however, coating technology is so far advanced that structure mottle in modern screens is negligible. Occasionally it is possible to have two screens with similar mottle characteristics. When this occurs there is a tendency for one to reinforce the other; in this case the mottle may become obtrusive.

RECIPROCITY

The *reciprocity law* states that:

> **The amount of density produced on a film is dependent only on the total amount of light energy employed.**

This means that if the exposure (E) remains constant, then the amount of density produced will also remain constant (all other factors being equal). Exposure is the product of Intensity (I) and Time (t):

$$E = It$$

If the reciprocity law holds true then, providing E is constant, any combination of I and t may be used to produce the same density. For example, if 100 'units' of E are required to produce a density of 1 then

$$
\left.
\begin{aligned}
E &= It \\
100 &= 10 \times 10 \\
&= 100 \times 1 \\
&= 1 \times 100 \\
&= 2 \times 50
\end{aligned}
\right\} \text{ All produce D = 1.0}
$$

and so on.

Reciprocity failure

That the simple relationship shown above (the reciprocity law) does not hold true, was proved by a researcher called Abney, who discovered that:

> **At very long or very short exposure times, the resulting density value was somewhat less than was expected.**

This means that the use of very high mA and short exposure times, or very low mA and long exposure times, will not produce the same result in terms of density as a set of exposure factors between the two extremes. In practice, reciprocity failure seems at a minimum for times of 0.1 s and is so small as to be insignificant for exposure times between about 0.002 s and 3 s.

There are a number of ways of illustrating reciprocity failure; one of the most common is to plot speed variation against exposure time (Fig. 5.19). As may be seen in the figure, a decrease in speed indicates reciprocity failure, as decreasing speed would give lower densities for a given amount of exposure.

Different films have differing reciprocity characteristics. Figure 5.20 illustrates the two extremes encountered in radiographic departments. Film directly exposed to X- or gamma radiation shows little or no variation in speed, while the monitor photography film shows no speed loss at short exposure times but some loss at longer exposure times. From this it can be deduced that to a large extent, reciprocity characteristics can be controlled in emulsion manufacture.

Finally, it is interesting to note that it is possible, with the aid of an engineer, to calibrate the mA settings of the X-ray set to hide the effects of selecting high or low mA values, providing that the timer is known to be accurate. This would apparently make the reciprocity law hold true.

SCREEN ASYMMETRY

This is a feature of some manufacturers' screens: it involves the provision of pairs of screens (i.e. front and back screens) which must be attached to the front and back of the cassette:

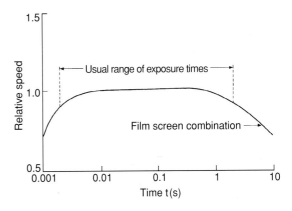

Fig. 5.19 Reciprocity failure: diagrammatic representation only.

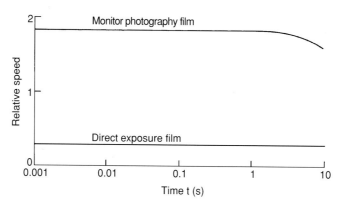

Fig. 5.20 Examples of reciprocity characteristics: diagrammatic only (actual data available from manufacturers).

The back screen may be slightly faster than the front to produce equal density on both sides of the film.

If the two screens in a cassette are identical, then the screen closest to the X-ray tube absorbs a proportion of the arriving X-ray beam and produces a certain amount of light. The back screen does not receive as many X-ray quanta, due to the fact some have already been absorbed, and therefore the amount of light output will be less. The front screen therefore produces a higher density on the film than the back screen. In order to counter this asymmetric production of density, the back screen is made slightly faster, so that even though it receives fewer X-ray quanta, its light output is the same as the front screen, thus producing the same density on both sides of the emulsion. This is normally achieved by the back screen having a slightly thicker coating of phosphor.

In calcium tungstate systems this asymmetry was of little practical significance. However, with the highly X-ray absorbent rare earth systems it has taken on some degree of importance. Failure to mount the screens in the cassette in the correct order can lead to significant speed reduction compared to that expected. However, it should be noted that not all screens are supplied in this front, back combination.

SPECTRAL EMISSION

Matching spectral output

The following subsections deal with the wavelengths of light (i.e. the colours) that are emitted by the various commonly used screen phosphors. It is important to match the spectral output of the screen to the spectral sensitivity of the film. In general, failure to do this will result in a loss of system speed and a loss of information transfer from the emergent beam from the patient to the film. However, occasionally a deliberate mismatch of screen and film sensitivity is used in order to reduce system speed and improve image quality. This is a particular feature of the rare earth film/screen systems and is more fully discussed below.

Calcium tungstate ($CaWO_4$)

This has been the commonly used phosphor for intensifying screens up until recent history. Calcium tungstate requires no activator and produces a continuous spectrum principally in the blue part of the visible spectrum, with a peak output at approximately 425 nm. Figure 5.21 illustrates the spectral output of the phosphor; superimposed on the same figure is the sensitivity of conventional monochromatic ('blue') film. As can be seen the film is sensitive to the majority of the screen output and therefore records all but a small proportion of the available information.

Rare earths

The elements known as rare earths are neither rare nor earths. They are soft, malleable metals and not at all in short supply. Cerium, the most abundant, is more plentiful than tin or lead.

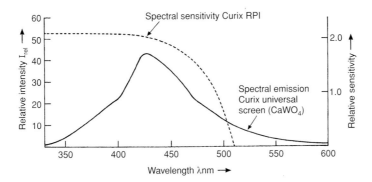

Fig. 5.21 Spectral sensitivity: Agfa-Gevaert Curix RPI film. Spectral emission: Agfa-Gevaert Curix Universal (CaWO₄) screen.

Thulium, the scarcest, is only slightly rarer than iodine. The misnomer arose because their oxides were at first taken for the elements themselves.

At an atomic level, all the 15 rare earths have two outer electrons, and in the penultimate shell they have eight or nine electrons. Their greatest difference is in the N shell. In atoms, this difference is very minute and so we find that the rare earths form a very close family. A mineral containing one of them contains all the others.

The rare earths are so nearly identical that separating them can involve thousands of steps. Because of this the individual elements did not become available until the late 1950s. However, the family has been used industrially since the early 1900s in the form of naturally occurring mixtures. Additionally, they are used in the phosphors of television cameras and in advanced technology lasers.

The following rare earths are those most commonly found in phosphors used in radiology:

Lanthanum (La)

- Atomic no. 57
- Atomic weight 138.91
- Electron configuration 2, 8, 18, 9, 2.

Lanthanum is highly reactive because it gives glass special light-bending properties, it is also used in expensive camera lenses. Lanthanum is involved in many rare earth screen phosphor patents.

Europium (Eu)

- Atomic no. 63
- Atomic weight 151.96
- Electron configuration 2, 8, 18, 25, 8, 2.

Europium is the most reactive rare earth. Atom for atom, europium can absorb more neutrons than any other element. This factor makes it very valuable for nuclear reactor control rods. In intensifying screens it is one of the principal activators.

Gadolinium (Gd)

- Atomic no. 64
- Atomic weight 157.25
- Electron configuration 2, 8, 18, 25, 9, 2.

From the mineral gadolinite, gadolinium comes in the middle of the rare earth series and divides the lighter metals, which impart pliancy to alloys, from the heavier strengthening metals. It is the principal element in many orthochromatic ('green') screen systems.

Terbium (Tb)

- Atomic no. 65
- Atomic weight 158.92
- Electron configuration 2, 8, 18, 26, 9, 2.

Terbium's principal use in screens is as an activator.

Yttrium (Y)

- Atomic no. 39
- Atomic weight 88.905
- Electron configuration 2, 8, 18, 9, 2.

Yttrium is not a rare earth but is a first transition metal, it is included because it has been used as an activator in some rare earth phosphor combinations.

Rare earth spectral emission

All the rare earth phosphors used in intensifying screens produce a line spectrum, the position and intensity of each line being dependent on the type and amount of dopant (i.e. activator) that has been added to the mother crystal. Conventionally the activator is written after the main phosphor formula and following a full stop, e.g. terbium-activated lanthanum oxybromide is written LaOBr.Tb. Somewhat conveniently, they can be divided into those that are suitable for use with orthochromatic ('green') sensitive film and those that are used with monochromatic ('blue') sensitive film. Table 5.2 illustrates three of the main phosphors. It should be noted that whilst not strictly a rare earth, barium fluorochloride has a rare earth activator.

As with calcium tungstate, it is vital to match the peak spectral lines with peak spectral sensitivity of the film to ensure maximum speed and information transfer. Figures 5.22, 5.23 and 5.24 show the spectral emission of lanthanum oxybromide (LaOBr.Tb), gadolinium oxysulphide (Gd_2O_2S.Tb) and barium fluorochloride (BaFCl.Eu) along with a film of suitable sensitivity superimposed on the same diagram.

The line emissions of the true rare earth phosphors extend throughout the whole of the visible spectrum (i.e. LaOBr.Tb emits both green and red light), but only the most intense (i.e. the blue) lines are recorded by the film.

A similar situation exists for Gd_2O_2S.Tb which has its highest light output in the green part of the spectrum with only a small light output in the blue. It is this factor that allows a mismatch of film and screens to produce an image even though the system will have low speed due to the relatively low intensity of the non-predominant spectral lines.

Also, it will be seen that the BaFCl.Eu phosphor produces essentially a continuous spectrum, with its peak in the ultraviolet at about 385 nm.

A close examination of the lanthanum and gadolinium spectra will reveal that the spectral lines of each are roughly at the same wavelengths, the variation being in the relative intensity of each spectral line. The intensity of each line is controlled by the amount and type of dopant. In general, increasing the concentration of dopant

Table 5.2 Rare earth screens: principal phosphors, symbols, emissions

Phosphor name	Formula.activator	Principal emission
Lanthanum oxybromide	LaOBr.Tb	Blue
Gadolinium oxysulphide	Gd_2O_2S.Tb	Green
Barium fluorochloride	BaFCl.Eu	Ultraviolet

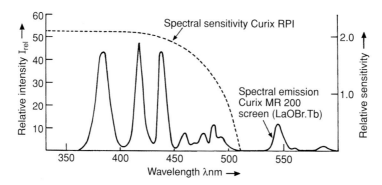

Fig. 5.22 Spectral sensitivity: Agfa-Gevaert Curix RPI film. Spectral emission: Agfa-Gevaert Curix MR200 (LaOBr.Tb) screen.

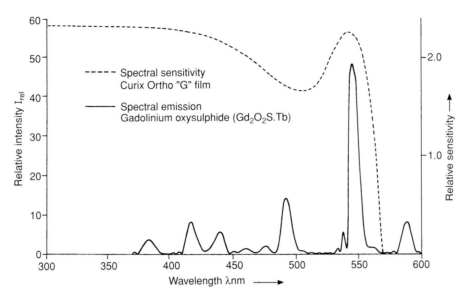

Fig. 5.23 Spectral sensitivity: Agfa-Gevaert Curix Ortho G film. Spectral emission: gadolinium oxysulphide (Gd$_2$O$_2$S.Tb).

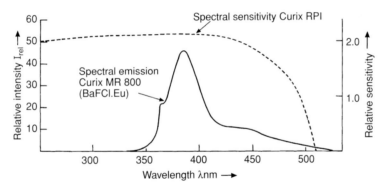

Fig. 5.24 Spectral sensitivity: Agfa-Gevaert Curix RPI film. Spectral emission: Agfa-Gevaert Curix MR800 (BaFCl.Eu) screen.

alters the peak emission towards the red end of the spectrum. Consequently there is no reason why LaOBr.Tb cannot be used to produce green-emitting screens providing the amount of terbium dopant present is high enough. However, in practice this is not done as it has a detrimental effect on overall efficiency. The same is also true of the gadolinium phosphors.

KILOVOLTAGE RESPONSE

The speed of all screens is to some extent kV dependent. Even the speed of calcium tungstate

screens alters with changing kV; however, in this case, the change in speed is so small as to be negligible for all practical purposes.

This does not apply to the rare earth screens. Figure 5.25 is a plot of relative speed versus kVp for four different speed classes, ranging from a calcium tungstate class 100 to a barium fluorochloride class 800 system. This shows peak speed for the rare earth systems at 80–85 kVp, with a fall in speed down to 60–65 kVp and a sharp decline at kVp lower than 60.

Between 80 kVp and 105 kVp (approximately), speed is more or less constant, being followed by a decline after about 105 kVp.

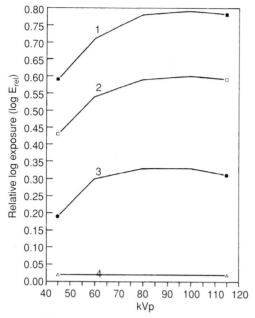

1. Speed class 800 (BaFCl.Eu)
2. Speed class 400 (LaOBr.Tb)
3. Speed class 200 (LaOBr.Tb)
4. Speed class 100 (CaWO$_4$)

Fig. 5.25 kV response rare earth screens.

In order to obtain the best use of the speed offered by rare earth screens, careful selection of the appropriate kV factors is necessary.

OTHER INFORMATION

Table 5.3 gives a comparison of the relative values of absorption, conversion, specific weight, phosphor thickness and efficiency for various phosphors.

CARE, CLEANING AND TESTING

These items are fully covered in Chapter 10, Quality assurance and tests.

SUMMARY

Crossover to cleaning

- *Crossover* causes a reduction in image quality and is caused by light which is not absorbed in the first emulsion layer passing through the base and exposing the second emulsion layer. It varies from 15 to 60%, depending on the systems in use (see Fig. 5.17).

- *Resolution* is a definite quantitative value and is measured in line pairs per millimetre (lp mm^{-1}). It defines the smallest object, or distance between two objects, that must exist if they are to be recorded as separate entities. Film/screen combinations have resolution ranges from 2 to 15 lp mm^{-1} (approximately).

- *Mottle* is the apparent granular appearance in areas of 'even' density on the film. There are three contributing factors: film grain, quantum mottle and structure mottle. Quantum mottle has the largest influence on this granular appearance.

- The *reciprocity law* says that the amount of density produced will be constant providing the exposure reaching the film is constant. The law fails, however, for very long or very short exposure times. *Reciprocity law failure* means that the density produced is less than expected.

Table 5.3	Phosphor data			
	Ortho	Blue	UV	Blue
	Gd$_2$O$_2$S.Tb	LaOBr.Tb	BaFCl.Eu	CaWO$_4$
% Absorption 80 kV	40.5	43.5	39.0	26.7
% Conversion	18.0	17.0	16.0	5
Specific weight	7.4	6.2	4.6	6.8
Phosphor thickness (μ)	207	288	347	250
Efficiency	7.3	7.4	6.2	1.7

- *Screen asymmetry* occurs when both screens in a cassette are identical. The back screen receives slightly less exposure than the front screen and therefore has a lower light output and contributes less to film exposure. In fast rare earth systems this can be a significant problem, therefore manufacturers sometimes provide screens in matched pairs, one marked front and the other back. The back screen is slightly faster, to balance the fact that it receives less exposure.

- The *colour of the light output* from screens must be matched to the peak spectral sensitivity of the film. This ensures maximum system speed and maximum information transfer. Occasionally a deliberate mismatch of screen output and film sensitivity is used in special cases.

- *Calcium tungstate* produces a continuous spectrum with a peak light output at about 425 nm (blue) and is used with *monochromatic film* (see Fig. 5.21).

- The *rare earth phosphors* produce a linetype spectrum with the major peaks in either the green or blue parts of the visible spectrum. The position of these peaks depends on the phosphor and dopant being used. Three of the most common phosphors are lanthanum oxybromide, gadolinium oxysulphide (both terbium-activated) and barium fluorochloride, europium-activated.
  Green-emitting phosphors are usually used with *orthochromatic* films (Figs 5.22, 5.23, 5.24).

- The speed of all phosphors is to some extent dependent on the kV used during the exposure. Rare earth phosphors are particularly *kV-dependent* in terms of their speed (Fig. 5.25).

- Screens should only be cleaned using the manufacturer's recommended materials and techniques.

REFERENCES

Penguin Dictionary of Science and Physics 1979
Product information from Agfa Gevaert Ltd, 27 Great West
    Road, Brentford, Middlesex TW8 9AX

Chapter 6
Photochemistry

INTRODUCTION

A knowledge of photochemistry does not have to draw on complex formulae or physical principles; it can be gained with logical reference to just a few simple chemical ideas.

For convenience, the subject of photochemistry can be divided into five sections:

1. The latent image and its formation
2. Development process
3. Fixation process
4. Washing
5. Silver conservation.

All these topics are highly interrelated, not only with one another but also with the chemistry of the film emulsion, the required sensitometric characteristics of the film and the automatic processor.

THE FORMATION OF THE LATENT IMAGE

The production of the latent image is the first stage of the photochemical process. It is here that all the information eventually seen is recorded as minute changes in the silver bromide crystal. These changes are so small that even an electron microscope reveals no difference between an exposed crystal and an unexposed crystal, and only development will show which is which. Even with modern computer techniques of image manipulation, if the information is not in the latent image, no amount of further 'processing' will increase or reveal more detail, although it may improve certain areas of particular interest.

Definition of latent image

The literal meaning of latent is 'hidden'. However, 'hidden image' is inadequate as a definition of 'latent image', which is more accurately defined as:

The image produced on the film after exposure but prior to development.

The exposure need not be useful exposure, as in the production of a radiography; it may be from any source that is sufficient to produce the minute changes within the silver bromide crystal necessary to render the crystal developable.

An understanding of latent image formation gives:

- A full understanding of the development and fixation process

- A better appreciation of the factors governing quality, for example resolution, basic fog, etc.

- An increased appreciation of the effects of X-radiation and light in relation to exposure and the final result.

Emulsion and silver bromide

The emulsion is a suspension of silver bromide and certain impurities in gelatine. In the laboratory, silver bromide is made in the following reaction:

$$AgNO_3 + KBr \rightarrow AgBr + KNO_3$$

i.e., silver nitrate + potassium bromide gives silver bromide + potassium nitrate.

The silver bromide produced in this way is what is known as a univalent ionic cubical lattice (Fig. 6.1). It has a structure similar to that of common salt, and after the initial formation of the cube shape grows simply by the addition of further ions of silver and bromine (i.e. Ag^+ ions and Br^- ions).

If this reaction is carried out in light the silver bromide immediately dissociates, turning the solution black (the silver bromide has effectively been exposed). Also the perfect crystal formed in this process is of no use photographically, as it exhibits none of the properties necessary for the formation of the latent image. In practice, therefore, the reaction is carried out in the gelatine suspension medium with excess amounts of potassium bromide.

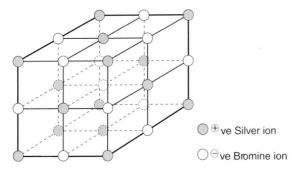

Fig. 6.1 Cubical silver bromide crystal lattice.

In practice:

$$AgNO_3 + KBr \text{ (excess)} \rightarrow AgBr + KNO_3$$
$$\text{In gelatine} \qquad \text{Suspended in gelatine}$$

(Reaction carried out in total darkness)

Effects of gelatine

Gelatine is obtained from the skins of dead animals, and occasionally from ligaments and bones, by the hydrolysis of the collagen fibres that are present in such skins. These fibres possess four principal features that are important in the formation of the latent image:

Chemical impurities

Photographic quality gelatine has had all the impurities removed from it before it reaches the production stage. However, this purification removes not only useless substances but also very useful ones. These useful substances are compounds of sulphur which form silver sulphides (AgS) and produce 'active' areas within the silver bromide crystals. It is therefore necessary to carefully add controlled amounts of sulphur to give the film its required latent image characteristics.

Physical defects in the crystal lattice structure

These are very significant in the production of the latent image, as they establish so-called electron traps within the lattice structure (see below).

Provides suitable growth medium

The reaction for the production of silver bromide is carried out in gelatine. Gelatine has the property of being able to keep separate the forming and growing nuclei of silver bromide, thus allowing crystals to grow without impinging on each other. This allows fine control of emulsion grain size.

Suspension and binder agent

Gelatine also acts as a suspension and binding agent for silver bromide when it is coated onto the film base and, fortunately, is totally inert even with prolonged storage. It is also thought that it prevents re-association of the silver and bromide ions released by exposure.

Electron traps

These are the main factors involved in latent image production, and they consist of areas of 'low energy' within the crystal lattice. Initially they are termed 'shallow', but they can be 'deepened' by various means and this deepening can be significant in the later stages of the latent image process.

'Shallow' traps are of two kinds:

- *Neutral colloids from impurities.* These have two effects, as they:
    Deepen electron traps, thus increasing stability in the early stages of image formation
    Consume certain photo by-products.

- *Defects in crystal lattice.* These defects, called kinks and jogs, are areas of crystal lattice fracture where the full bonding potential between two ions is not used but stored between two or

more points (as in Fig. 6.2). They are mainly formed by growing crystals coming into contact with each other. This produces forces within the crystal lattice causing the crystals to break up and produce 'free' lattice chains. These free chains possess ions that are not completely neutralised by their opposite ion and attempt to share their charge with adjacent points on the structure (point 'b' in Fig. 6.2). At this point the electrical potential of the crystal differs and an area of 'low energy' is produced. There are many such areas in a single crystal and these are the most significant factors in electron trap production.

Effects of excess potassium bromide

The reaction to produce silver bromide is carried out in excess potassium bromide. This produces two main beneficial effects:

- *Alters crystal shapes*: This has the advantage of producing more crystal defects and consequently more electron traps.

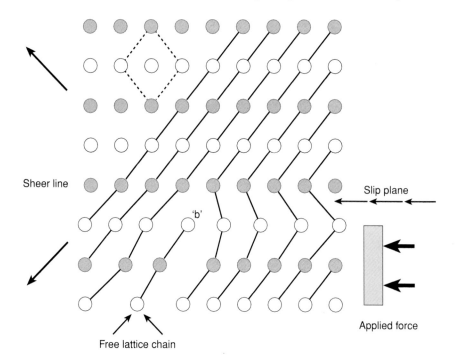

Fig. 6.2 Production of crystal lattice defects.

- *Increases surface barrier of individual crystals.* This surface potential barrier is produced to protect individual crystals against unselective developers and certain other by-products of exposure and processing. It consists of a barrier of bromine ions (Br^-) that collect at the surface of the crystal. Excessive potassium bromide ensures an adequate supply of these ions as the crystal is formed.

Free interstitial silver ions

These are positively charged silver ions that are trapped within the crystal during its formation. The presence of these ions is not obvious from the simple equation; however, their presence is vital for two main reasons:

- First, they provide the free silver that is necessary during the early stages of latent image formation
- Second, they assist the balancing of the negatively charged bromine ion barrier, thereby ensuring the silver bromide crystal is electrically neutral.

They are also free to migrate around the crystal, and this ability to travel assists in the formation of the latent sub-image centre (see next section).

MECHANISMS OF LATENT IMAGE FORMATION

The actual way in which the latent image forms falls into the all-too-frequent category of 'no one really knows what happens but we do know how altering various components alters the end result'. Bearing this in mind, there are two main theories of formation:

- Gurney Mott (classical) theory
- Mitchell (modern) theory.

All other theories, of which there are many, broadly fall into one of these two catagories.

Both the Gurney Mott theory and the Mitchell theory are based on the partial reduction of silver bromide crystals during exposure. This partial reduction is achieved by the free interstitial silver ions (Ag^+) gaining an electron from some source (usually exposure to light, X-rays or both).

Effects of exposure

The desired result of exposure as far as the latent image is concerned is the release of an electron within the silver bromide crystals lattice. Exposure of any substance to a source containing the correct wavelengths and energy produces three effects:

1. Compton effect
2. Photoelectric effect
3. Pair production.

In the X-ray to blue range (1 – 430 nm) used to expose conventional unsensitised (monochromatic) film, only the first two effects – the Compton effect and the photoelectric effect – occur in the silver bromide crystal. Of these two, the photoelectric effect predominates, as silver bromide is an ionic compound and has very few of the unbound electrons that are necessary for the Compton effect to occur. Approximately 96% of the electrons produced are from the photoelectric effect. In any case, both effects release a high kinetic energy electron that can be used in latent image formation. Unfortunately, not all these electrons remain useful.

Energy of the released electrons

The energy of the electrons released by exposure is important, as to be useful in image formation they must be able to enter the conduction band of the silver bromide crystal.

This band is one of the following three energy bands that exist in metallic crystalline solids:

1. Valency band
2. Forbidden gap
3. Conduction band.

The three bands can be represented as an energy level diagram (as in Fig. 6.3).

Valency band. This is the range of energies that may occur in the outer electrons of an atom. They allow the electron to take part in ionic or covalent bonding. If the electrons in the outer shells are within this energy band they may be

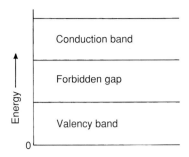

Fig. 6.3 Energy level diagram.

useful in forming bonds with other atoms and may form a new compound.

Forbidden gap. In order to enter the conduction band, electrons must traverse the forbidden gap. This is a range of energies that are not allowable according to the theories of wave mechanics. Those with enough energy pass through and become 'free electrons' within the crystal and are available to form the latent image. Those with insufficient energy eventually fall back into an orbit.

Conduction band. If an electron has a certain range of energies it can exist within this band and may be available to form the latent image. This does not alter the electronic configuration of the atom but, providing it retains the range of allowed energies, moves as a free electron within the crystal.

An electron that is successful in entering the conduction band leaves a 'gap' in a higher orbit of the atom concerned in the initial interaction. This gap is called a 'hole' and is effectively a unit of positive charge. The hole would make the structure of the crystal 'unstable', but the migration of a colloidal sulphur particle to the site renders the hole ineffective.

THEORIES OF LATENT IMAGE FORMATION

As stated previously, there are two principal theories of latent image formation: the Gurney Mott and the Mitchell. Both theories suggest that it is a two-stage process involving *nucleation* and *growth*, and while both have general agreement on the growth process, they differ on the mechanism of the nucleation process.

Gurney Mott theory

Nucleation

This is best described by a diagram (Fig. 6.4) showing the various stages involved.

Stage one. An electron that has been released by exposure is captured by a trapping centre and temporarily held. A mobile, positively charged silver ion may migrate to this centre and form a silver atom, but . . .

Stage two. Before the arrival of this silver ion, the electron may escape from the trap due to its vibrational energy and again become free in the conduction band. Eventually it becomes trapped long enough to be joined by a silver ion giving a silver atom . . .

Stage three. Unfortunately, a single silver atom is unstable, separation occurs and stages one and two happen again.

Stage four. Fortunately, during its short life the single silver atom can act as a trap for another electron, and if another silver ion is attracted to this site . . .

Stage five. A stable two-atom silver speck, called a *latent sub-image centre*, is formed. This then grows as detailed later.

Mitchell theory

Nucleation

As for the Gurney Mott theory, this is best described by the use of a diagram (Fig. 6.5).

Stages one and two. A free silver ion comes near to a shallow electron trap and deepens it. While this trap is deepened, a free electron, released by exposure, and another free silver ion approach the trap together and immediately form a silver atom. This is called a pre-image centre.

Stage three. Unfortunately, as in the Gurney Mott theory, the single silver atom is unstable and it dissociates into a silver ion and an electron.

Stages four and five. Stages one and two recur. During its life the single silver atom does not act as a trap for a further electron (as in the Gurney Mott theory) but must acquire a second silver ion. If it is successful and an electron arrives before the escape of this second silver ion, a stable *latent sub-image centre* forms.

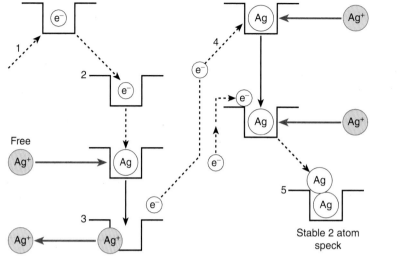

Fig. 6.4   Diagrammatic representation of the Gurney Mott theory.

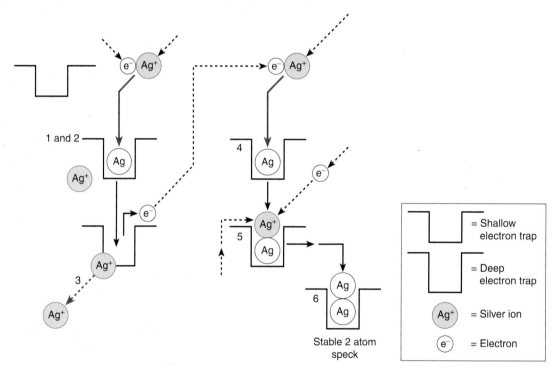

Fig. 6.5   Diagrammatic representation of the Mitchell theory.

Growth

There is, fortunately, general agreement on the growth process. Both the Gurney Mott and Mitchell theories consider that this is due to the deepening of the electron traps, because of the presence of the latent sub-image centre, increasing the attraction of that site compared to the shallow trap.

The increasing electrical attraction of these points in the crystal attracts the electrons from exposure and the silver ions from the crystal lattice, or from the supply of free interstitial ions, causing a build-up of silver atoms.

Many sub-image centres are formed throughout the crystal on one single exposure, but growth does proceed in a preferential way as the first formed sub-image centres tend to exhibit greater electrical attraction. During their growth, the ever-enlarging silver specks start to invade the surface of the crystal. This reduces the surface potential barrier (Fig. 6.6) by destroying the crystal lattice in the area, therefore rendering the crystal more susceptible to development.

When growth is complete, the sub-image centres are commonly called *development centres*.

ACTION OF DEVELOPER ON SILVER BROMIDE CRYSTALS

The function of developer is to reduce the exposed silver bromide crystals to metallic silver. This function is performed by the donation of electrons in a selective fashion (see Selectivity, p. 100). No developer is completely selective and therefore a developing agent that reduces exposed crystals quickly is used. The exposed crystals have a gap in the surface potential barrier, therefore allowing electrons from the developer easier access (see Fig. 6.6) to perform this reduction.

The use of excess potassium bromide in the production of the crystal increases the surface potential barrier, thereby assisting the process of selectivity.

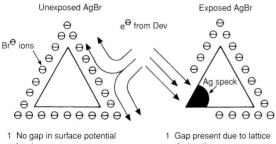

1 No gap in surface potential barrier
2 Electrons have difficulty penetrating

1 Gap present due to lattice destruction
2 Electrons penetrate easily
3 Crystal converted quickly

Fig. 6.6 Effect of the bromine ion barrier.

SUMMARY

• The production of the *latent image* is the first stage of the photochemical process. It is defined as the image produced on the film after exposure but prior to development. Changes produced after exposure in the silver bromide crystals of the emulsion are so small that even an electron microscope cannot reveal them.

• Film emulsion is a suspension of *silver bromide in gelatine*; pure silver bromide is a cube-shaped crystal lattice (see Fig. 6.1). However, this crystal is of no use photographically, as it has none of the properties required to obtain a latent image.

• *Gelatine* is vital to the production of the latent image because it provides:

  Chemical impurities
  These consist mainly of sulphur and produce 'active' areas in the silver bromide crystal
  Physical defects in crystal lattice structure.
  These are most probably the most important factors in the latent image production, as they introduce electron traps (see below)
  Growth medium
  Allows silver bromide crystals to grow during the chemical reaction
  Suspension and binding agent
  It is used to coat the emulsion onto the film base.

• *Electron traps* within the crystal are areas of low energy that are caused by lattice defects and impurities from the gelatine. They are significant because it is in these areas that, after exposure, the latent image starts to form (see Fig. 6.2). Also it will be noticed that there is an *excess of potassium bromide* used in the emulsion production. This has two beneficial effects:

— It alters crystal shapes, giving more electron traps
— It increases the surface potential barrier of the crystal, thus improving selectivity (see Fig. 6.6).

- During the production of the emulsion, *free interstitial silver ions* are contained within the silver bromide crystal and provide the free silver that is necessary during the early stages of latent image formation.

- There are two main theories of latent image formation: *Gurney Mott* and *Mitchell*:

  — Both make use of the electrons that are released in the crystal due to exposure, and the fact that these electrons may become free in the conduction band of the crystal
  — Once the electrons released by exposure become free electrons, they eventually combine with a silver ion to produce a silver atom at an electron trap, and
  — A latent sub-image centre, which grows by attracting more silver atoms until it becomes a development centre
  — The process of combination of silver ions and electrons is called nucleation
  — The enlargement of the sub-image centre is known as growth
  — The first formed latent sub-image centre tends to become the largest because of its greater electrical attraction
  — Growth also causes the breakdown of the crystal lattice structure, which allows entry of the developer electrons
  — Entry is easier than in the unexposed crystal (see Fig. 6.6) and helps with the selectivity of the developer, i.e. its ability to distinguish between exposed and unexposed crystals.

- The mechanics of latent image formation are still only theory; the actual process is still not fully understood.

DEVELOPERS AND FIXERS

Developer and fixer chemistry depend a great deal on the ability to understand and apply the concept of pH.

THE CONCEPT OF pH

pH is a quantitative method of measuring the degree of acidity or alkalinity of a solution.

It is based on the fact that concentrations of ions that coexist in solution may be described by a number called the equilibrium constant:

Equilibrium constant = concentration of products in a chemical reaction/concentration of reactants.

Pure water is chosen as the basis of the pH scale. Under normal conditions this is very slightly ionised into H^+ ions and OH^- ions and has a specially named equilibrium constant (Kw) called the ion product of water. This is equal to the product of $[H^+][OH^-]$ and has the value of 10^{-14} at 25°C, i.e.:

$$Kw = [H^+][OH^-] = 10^{-14}$$

The square brackets are used to indicate that concentrations are being considered and the mol/l is a method of measuring these concentrations.

The acid 'portion' of a substance in solution is the H^+ ion content, while the alkaline portion is the OH^- ion content. Distilled water is neither acid nor alkaline, therefore these ions are present in equal concentrations. From the above equa-

Table 6.1 Hydrogen ion concentrations and related pH values

	[H+] (mole/litre)	pH
	1 or 10^0	0
	0.1 or 10^{-1}	1
	0.01 or 10^{-2}	2
Increasing acidity	0.001 or 10^{-3}	3
	0.0 001 or 10^{-4}	4
	0.00 001 or 10^{-5}	5
	0.000 001 or 10^{-6}	6
Pure water	0.0 000 001 or 10^{-7}	7
	0.00 000 001 or 10^{-8}	8
	0.000 000 001 or 10^{-9}	9
Increasing alkalinity	0.0 000 000 001 or 10^{-10}	10
	0.00 000 000 001 or 10^{-11}	11
	0.000 000 000 001 or 10^{-12}	12
	0.0 000 000 000 001 or 10^{-13}	13
	0.00 000 000 000 001 or 10^{-14}	14

tion it can be seen that the ion product of both H^+ and OH^- is 10^{-14}; as they are present in equal proportions, there must be 10^{-7} mol/l of H^+ ions and 10^{-7} mol/l of OH^- ions.

Acid solutions are those with H^+ ion concentrations greater than 10^{-7} mol/l, while alkaline solutions have a H^+ ion concentration of less than 10^{-7} mol/l. This is demonstrated in Table 6.1.

As the manipulation of such figures proved to be inconvenient, a simpler method was devised; this states that 'pH is the log of the reciprocal of the hydrogen ion concentration'. This removes the large number of zeros in the values and the negative value of the power:

$$pH = \log_{10}\frac{1}{\left[H^+\right]}$$

Therefore, pH is in the range 0–14.

Developers

Most developers for automatic processing have a pH range of 9.6–10.6, and to work to optimum efficiency must be maintained within $\pm\,0.2$ of the manufacturer's recommended value, otherwise detrimental effects may occur to the final image quality, thus reducing diagnostic information (Fig. 6.7).

Fixers

Fixers for automatic processing have a pH range of 4.2–4.9, and again must be maintained at the recommended value to work efficiently. If allowed to rise above 4.9 they will still perform fixation, but problems will arise with the hardener present in modern fixers, causing transportation difficulties in the processor and eventually destroying the solution (Fig. 6.7).

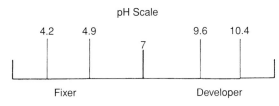

Fig. 6.7 The pH scale and its range for developers and fixers.

SUMMARY

- pH is a measure of the degree of acidity or alkalinity of a solution
- Its value is the log of the reciprocal of the hydrogen ion concentration of a solution
- A pH value of 7 is neutral
- Higher than 7 is alkali
- Lower than 7 is acid
- As pH is a log scale, small changes in value are large changes in ion concentration.

DEVELOPERS

Some of the terms used in this section are defined in Chapter 8 (Sensitometry).

All conventional radiographic emulsions are subject contrast amplifiers when correctly processed:

- They have an average gradient that is greater than 1, usually between 1.8 and 3.5.

- The chemistry of the emulsion and the developer are arranged so that these limits are available over a wide range of different conditions.

X-ray developers are considered to be high speed, and have the ability to produce an image in approximately 20 seconds, thereby enabling 90-second processing:

- This speed is mainly due to working at high temperatures, but unfortunately this tends to increase the base + fog level of the film.

- In order to reduce this, a move to 2- and 3-minute processing would have to be made.

- A base + fog level of less than 0.2 is desirable, but this is problematic, for the reasons outlined above.

Developer must:

- Produce a maximum density of 3.0–4.0.

- Contain additives that allow the emulsion to be transported through high speed, high temperature roller processing.

- Contain additives that absorb detrimental by-products of the developer action as well as guarding against auto-oxidation and the non-uniform nature of water supplies (this allows solutions to be used for long periods without excessive maintenance or replenishment).

- Be capable of being stored for long periods in a wide range of conditions without undesirable effects, when in concentrated solutions.

- Contain chemicals that are as non-hazardous as possible, to conform with health and safety regulations.

- Be simple to use.

Functions

For a chemical to be a developer it must possess two main properties, conversion and selectivity.

Conversion

The chemical must be able to precipitate metallic silver from the silver salts of bromide, chloride and iodide or combinations of these salts. (Fig. 6.8)

The most common silver halide in X-ray emulsions is silver bromide (AgBr). This is normally mixed with a small proportion of silver iodide (AgI) to produce an emulsion with the desired characteristics. The ratio is of the order of 96%

AgBr to 4% AgI. Figure 6.8 shows the reaction that occurs when AgBr is placed in a developing agent.

The developer reduces the AgBr to metallic silver and itself becomes oxidised, therefore developers are reducing agents. It can be seen that the desirable reaction has occurred. However, two by-products have also been formed, both of which adversely affect further development and must be combated by other agents (see Developer constituents, below). The developing agent donates electrons to the AgBr crystal during the reduction process.

Selectivity

This is the ability of a developing agent to differentiate between exposed silver halide and unexposed silver halide, changing only the exposed crystals to metallic silver.

Many chemicals are able to reduce AgBr to metallic silver but few have the property of selectivity. It is an unfortunate fact that even those used as developing agents are not completely selective. In practice, therefore, developers reduce exposed AgBr quicker than unexposed AgBr. This differential ability can be evaluated and is called the *selectivity ratio*. It is the difference in the rate between the development of exposed and unexposed grains of silver bromide. The ratio is high in selective developers and low

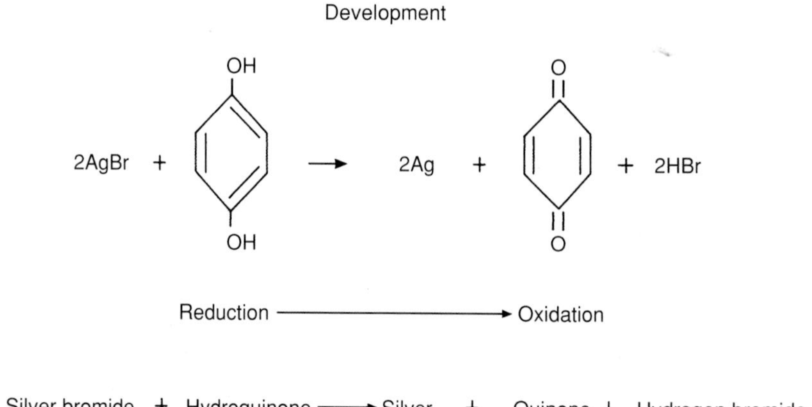

Development

Silver bromide + Hydroquinone ⟶ Silver + Quinone + Hydrogen bromide

Fig. 6.8 The chemical action of developer on silver bromide (simplified).

in unselective developers. Again, there are additions which may be made to developer solutions to try and improve this ratio. Usually, highly selective developers are slow acting whereas unselective developers are fast. In practice, a trade-off exists between speed and selectivity (see also Latent image, p. 91).

Amplification gain

It is this feature of the film, latent image and developer system that makes photography a viable proposition.

Amplification gain is a measure of the extent to which the developer increases the initial effect of exposure on the silver halide grains.

Many experiments have been carried out to assess the numerical value of this gain, giving results ranging from 10^6 to 10^{12}. However, the most widely accepted figure seems to be 10^9:

Ag + development = Amplification gain of 10^9

The photographic process is the only process known at this time which gives gains of this order. A close rival is a heat transfer process (Diazo), having a gain factor of about 10^3. To put this value in perspective, a sound system giving amplification of 10^9 would produce approximately 200 000 W. An average domestic system gives about 20–30 W.

DEVELOPING SOLUTIONS IN THE AUTOMATIC PROCESSOR

Automatic processing developers have special features that make them quite different from manual processing solutions. It is important, therefore, not to infer similar properties, and to realise that, due to advancements in technology, certain substances are given traditional names that are not strictly accurate in chemical definition.

In the following sections, reference will be made to 'machine tank developer' and 'developer replenisher'. These should be considered as separate entities, and care should be taken to

state which is being considered. The major difference between the two is shown in Table 6.2. In general, most have a pH in the range 9.6–10.6.

CONSTITUENTS

The constituents of developer replenisher and machine tank developer are shown in Table 6.2. It is important to remember that:

Developer replenisher + starter = machine tank developer.

The need for replenishment

Certain by-products of development affect its activity, and as development proceeds the developing agent is used up. As the developing agent is used up its concentration falls, and the developer becomes less active (exhausted). In a practical situation this would necessitate frequent changing of the developer to maintain consistent results, both from the image and the machine/mechanical point of view. In order to obviate this, a certain amount of replenisher is added to the machine tank every time a film is fed into the machine. The replenisher replaces the exhausted developer and maintains the concentration of the other active components at the

Table 6.2 The constituents of developer

Developer replenisher	Machine tank
1. Developing agent(s)	
2. Preservative	
3. Accelerator	
4. Restrainer	
5. Buffer	
6. Sequestering agent	
7. Solvent	+ 9. Starter solution
8. Other additions:	
Hardening agent	
Wetting agent	
Anti-frothant	
Fungicide	

correct levels. It also maintains the physical quantity of the solution in the tank.

The principal factors affecting developer replenishment are:

1. Area of film processed
2. Average density of the film
3. Silver content of the film
4. Maximum density required
5. Thickness of the emulsion
6. Single or duplitised coating
7. Processor work load
8. Amount of aerial oxidation.

Note: Many of the factors listed above are related to each other and decided by the film chemistry. However, knowledge of this data is essential to correctly replenish solutions, even though the manufacturer freely provides this information in the form of recommended replenishment rates.

Replenishment in most processors is usually governed by an average rate per length of film (for developer, the average rate is 40–60 ml for every 35 cm). This means that large films are actually receiving slight under-replenishment, whereas small film sizes receive over-replenishment, the net effect being that, over an average working day, replenishment is correct. However, most modern machines are capable of assessing actual film size and therefore replenish according to area. Some processors also calculate average density as well as area, giving even more accurate replenishment. This is achieved by a suitably programmed microprocessor (i.e. computer) which will also monitor all other automatic processor functions (see Ch. 7, Automatic processing).

Starter solution

In theory, once correctly set, replenishment could continue indefinitely; but emulsion flaking and dirt accumulation in the developer tank necessitate regular cleaning.

After draining and cleaning the main tank, fresh developer replenisher is added to fill the tank to the recommended level. If the rollers were replaced and a film developed, it would exhibit all the features shown in Figure 6.9.

The change in the characteristic curve is due to the high activity of replenisher. If films are still processed through this solution, its activity will eventually fall and balance at the correct level. This is due to the increase in bromine ion (Br^-) concentration and depression of the pH value, both of which are caused by development (Fig. 6.9). To enable immediate use of the processor, starter solution is added to the machine tank. This is a restrainer solution which adds weak acid and Br^- ions, therefore depressing activity to the required level before films are processed.

A certain quantity of starter solution is required for every mixed litre of developer replenisher solution to make machine tank developer. However, some manufacturers supply developer which contains starter solution and just requires mixing with water. Replenisher is then available separately.

Developing agents

There are two principal agents used in automatic processor developers:

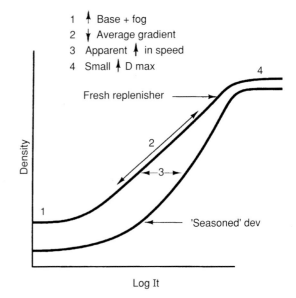

Fig. 6.9 The effect of processing a film in replenisher as compared to 'seasoned developer'.

Table 6.3 Characteristics of different developing agents

Developing agent	Characteristics
Common name: Phenidone (P) Chemical name: 1-phenyl-3-pyrazolidone Discovered by: Ilford Labs, 1940 Main modern use: General use	1. High speed 2. Low selectivity 3. Low contrast 4. Only 10–15% compared with Q to give similar activity 5. Activity not so dependent on Br⁻ concentration 6. Liquid concentrate
Common name: Hydroquinone (Q) Chemical name: para-dihydroxybenzene Discovered by: Sir W de W Abney, 1880 Main modern use: Graphic arts	1. High contrast 2. Slow speed 3. High selectivity 4. Susceptible to auto-oxidation 5. Activity very dependent on temperature and pH
Phenidone hydroquinone (PQ)	1. High speed 2. Higher contrast than Q 3. Low auto-oxidation rate 4. Not excessively Br⁻ ion dependent 5. Susceptible to pH variations 6. Temperature dependent 7. Superadditivity 8. Liquid concentrate 9. Less likely to cause dermatitis 10. Long shelf life

- Phenidone (P)
- Hydroquinone (Q).

P and Q are not used separately but in combination to produce a phenidone hydroquinone (PQ)-type developer. Some of the characteristics of P and Q, separately and combined, are listed in Table 6.3. The advantages of using two agents in combination are shown in Figure 6.10. As well as making full use of the superadditive effect, com-

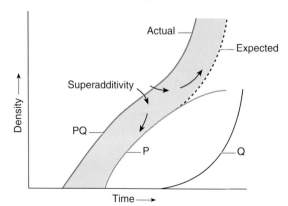

Fig. 6.10 Diagrammatic representation of superadditivity.

bining agents in this way enables the manufacturer to control base + fog, contrast, speed, etc. Correct replenishment removes most of the problems experienced with a PQ combination.

Superadditivity and regeneration

This is another almost unique effect of the photographic process. It is an advantage that arises when using agents in combination. Superadditivity (see Fig. 6.10) may be described as:

> **The combined activities of two developing agents in the same solution which is greater than the sum of their separate activities.**

It is still not completely clear how this mechanism functions, although it is believed to be due to:

- The relative size of the ionised form of the developing agents in the early stages of their effect on the sensitised AgBr crystal.

- Hydroquinone developers that contain sulphite (of which radiographic developers are a good example) form a first oxidation product of hydroquinone called hydroquinone monosulphonate. In the presence of phenidone this forms a superadditive system of great power.

- Regeneration. In this reaction the first oxidation product of phenidone reacts with hydroquinone to yield ordinary phenidone. This means that the concentration of the most active ingredient is kept high, thus assisting the left shift shown in Figure 6.10.

Advantages and disadvantages of phenidone hydroquinone (PQ) developers

Advantages. PQ developers have certain advantages – so much so that they are the only ones used for radiographic processing. This is because they:

- Have a more efficient superadditivity system
- Have a greater regeneration effect
- Are relatively cheap
- Can be made as liquid concentrates
- Have a long shelf life
- Have a long working life
- Are more active at equivalent pH values
- Enable the easy control of replenishment
- Are not susceptible to bromide ion concentrations
- Are less likely to cause contact dermatitis
- Are less likely to cause staining on clothes or hands
- Do not tend to have an unacceptable odour after prolonged use.

Disadvantages. Hydroquinone is classified as a hazardous chemical and therefore work has been underway to find a replacement to improve the relative safety of developer both to the person handling it and in terms of the environmental impact. As a result of this research, hydroquinone-free developers are now available where the chemical has been replaced with ascorbic acid (vitamin C).

Preservative

Developer activity is reduced by oxidation. This oxidation takes place in two ways:

- Normal development action (Fig. 6.8)
- Aerial or auto-oxidation.

Developing agents + oxygen → oxidised developing agents + OH^- ions.

The problem is aerial oxidation; if not reduced to a minimum, it soon produces coloured insoluble products which depress, and would eventually destroy, the activity of the developer. To reduce this aerial oxidation to an acceptable level, various forms of sulphite can be added to the developer solution.

Agent

The most common agent used in automatic processing developers is potassium metabisulphite. This is used, especially in liquid concentrate developers, because of its high solubility and greater preserving efficiency compared to other preserving agents (such as sodium sulphite).

Function

The active 'ingredient' is the sulphite ion. This forms sulphonates with early oxidation products. These sulphonates are colourless and inert and have two properties:

- They slow down formation of discoloured products
- They discourage oxidation.

A highly simplified view of how this works is to imagine that the sulphite combines with dissolved oxygen, in the developer solution and at the surface of the developer, to produce the sulphonates in solution. However, in practice it is not as simple as this, as it is not a case of preferential absorption of oxygen by the preserving agent.

Note: Potassium metabisulphite is acidic. However, this acidity is more than compensated for by the addition of sufficient alkali to counteract its effect and maintain the alkalinity of the developer.

Aerial oxidation is kept to a minimum in automatic processing by a combination of the following methods:

- High preservative level in the developer

- Floating lid in the developer replenisher tank to reduce the surface area of the developer in contact with the air

- Closely fitting rollers, again to reduce surface area in contact with the air

- Deep narrow tanks in the processor so that the surface area to volume is kept as small as possible

- Totally enclosed replenisher tanks when using automatic chemical mixers.

Accelerator

Developers are very pH dependent and must be alkaline to work effectively and produce the desired result. Unfortunately, neither hydroquinone nor phenidone are particularly alkaline, and if simply dissolved in water do not produce a working developer. Both agents require an activator to stimulate their developing properties. This activator is called the accelerator; it is alkali, which is added to the developer solution. The activity of the developer is closely controlled by varying the amount of accelerator present.

Agent

Automatic processing developers are considered to be highly active and therefore have a high amount of accelerator present. The agent used is either sodium or potassium hydroxide. Both these agents are strongly alkaline and are particularly useful in high contrast developers containing hydroquinone, as their high solubility makes them ideal for production as liquid concentrates.

Function

The accelerator controls developer activity by assuring correct pH value. It affects contrast and speed so that, in balance with other agents in the developer, the desired image quality is produced.

Restrainer (anti-foggant)

As stated previously, restrainer is added to replenisher to produce machine tank developer when starting the machine from 'dry'. In this case it is known as starter solution (see Starter solutions, p. 102).

However, restrainer is also present in normally prepared developer replenisher where it may be called an anti-foggant. It is therefore good practice to consider starter solution as additional restrainer.

Agent

There are two principal types of restraining agent in use:

- Organic restrainers, e.g. benzotriazole
- Inorganic restrainers, e.g. potassium bromide.

Developer replenisher uses an organic benzotriazole-type restrainer. This is principally because:

- Organic restrainers appear to be capable of restraining base + fog with little or no effect on film speed. This is not true of inorganic restrainers, which are occasionally deliberately used to control film speed during processing.

- With high speed developers, the amount of inorganic restrainer required to keep 'fog' within acceptable limits would be such that image staining may occur, as potassium bromide in large quantities is a silver bromide solvent.

Because of these features it is common to find organic benzotriazole used in developer replenisher, and potassium bromide plus acetic acid used in starter solution (see also Low temperature chemistry, p. 110).

Function

The function of the restrainer is to improve the selectivity of the developer, ensuring low fog and high image contrast. Its action is to increase the effective bromine ion barrier that exists around silver bromide crystals (see Latent image, p. 91). The barrier is increased around both exposed and unexposed crystals. However, exposed crystals have some crystal lattice destruction where the protection is useless (Fig. 6.11).

The amount of restrainer provided in developer is sufficient to give adequate protection of the crystals when the replenisher is used in the conventional manner. When starter is added (it will be recalled that there is some acetic acid present in this solution, as well as potassium bromide) this depresses the pH of the replenisher, thereby giving the correct activity. The potassium bromide provides the small additional amount of restrainer to give correct selectivity.

Buffer

Figure 6.8 shows how the development process releases bromine ions from the silver bromide complexes within the emulsion and hydrogen ions from the developing agent, due to the donation of electrons from, in this case, the hydroxyl groups in hydroquinone. These combine to form hydrogen bromide, but as this occurs in an aqueous solution it becomes hydrobromic acid. This by-product will depress the pH value of the developer solution and take it away from its ideal level. This affects the activity of the developer and if allowed to persist would render the developer useless.

Agent

A buffer is normally a solution of weak acid and alkali compounds, for example boric acid and sodium hydroxide.

Function

The *Penguin Dictionary of Science* defines a buffer as:

'a solution the hydrogen ion concentration of which, and hence its acidity or alkalinity, is practically unchanged by dilution, and which resists a change in pH on the addition of acid or alkali.'

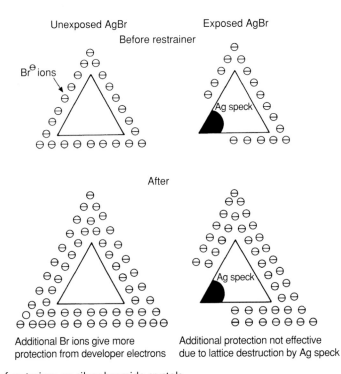

Unexposed AgBr   Exposed AgBr

Before restrainer

Br⁻ ions   Ag speck

After

Additional Br ions give more protection from developer electrons   Additional protection not effective due to lattice destruction by Ag speck

Fig. 6.11 The effect of restrainer on silver bromide crystals.

In the case of developers, it can be considered that this is achieved by the absorption of the hydrogen ions before they combine with the bromine ions. In fact the actual effect of the hydrobromic acid is limited by the equilibrium concentrations that are allowed by the equilibrium equation. This limits the number of free hydrogen and bromine ions available and therefore the amount of acid produced. A buffer helps maintain pH and therefore activity by absorbing harmful by-products of development action, while the preservative maintains activity by absorbing products of auto-oxidation.

Sequestering agent

This addition is used to counter the problems that may occur if hard water is used to make up developer solutions. It prevents the precipitation of calcium sludge which would otherwise show up as chalky deposits on the dry film or cause scaling of the developer tank. The scaling would be somewhat similar to lime scale found in domestic kettles.

The calcium sludge is caused by a reaction that takes place between the calcium and magnesium salts present in the water supply and the sodium sulphite compounds in the developer. Under normal conditions this does not present a problem as caustic alkali developers (i.e. X-ray developers) do not suffer from calcium precipitation. However, extremes do occur and sufficient sequestering agent is added to cope with even the hardest water supplies.

Agent

Sodium salt of ethylene diamine tetra-acetic acid (EDTA sodium salt).

Function

The function of this agent is to soften hard water supplies, thus preventing precipitation of the calcium and magnesium salts onto the surface of the film. This is achieved by transforming the calcium and magnesium salts into soluble complexes. These complexes are inert to the sulphite

components of the solution and, as a result, do not precipitate out.

Solvent

The solvent used in the photographic process is almost always water and normal tap water is more than adequate for use with conventional X-ray developers.

Advantages

- Relatively low cost and availability
- All the salts produced in the photographic process, with only one exception, are soluble in water.

This removes the need for any intermediate steps to remove deleterious by-products that complicate many other processes.

Disadvantage

- The water supply is not constant in character.

There are various problems associated with the non-constant nature of domestic and industrial water supplies. Table 6.4 itemises the major problem areas.

The most significant practical precaution that can be taken is the use of filtered water in the preparation of solutions. A large quantity of foreign material can be present in a filter that has been in use for even a short time.

OTHER ADDITIONS

It is the so-called other additions that principally distinguish developers for automatic processing and those for manual processing. However, commercially available solutions differ very little, whether for manual or automatic processing, and as these additional chemicals provide significant improvements to both manual and automatic processing situations, examination of actual formulae will probably reveal little difference between the two. There are four principal other additions:

Table 6.4 Problems associated with water supplies

Problem	Indication	Solution
Hard water	Excessive calcium + magnesium salts Chalky deposits on film	Sequestering agent: sufficient included for hardest water supplies
Excessive iron + copper content	Can cause fogging + oxidise developer (usually from copper pipes used to supply water to processor)	All specifications for installation of automatic processors now include the use of plastic pipes
Suspended solid matter	Particles of grit, dirt, etc., scratching of film in processor	Use of filtered water supply for mixing chemicals, usually from output side of water panel
Fluoride and chlorides	Added at water treatment works to control bacteria content	No photographic effects in concentrations usually present

1. Hardening agent
2. Wetting agent
3. Anti-frothant
4. Fungicide.

Hardening agent

Probably the worst situation in which to place the photographic emulsion (especially the gelatine used as the suspension agent for the silver bromide) is a warm aqueous alkaline solution. Developer is an excellent example of such a solution. The high temperatures in use can cause excessive swelling and softening of the emulsion, by encouraging water absorption. By controlling this effect the hardener reduces to a minimum the following problems:

- Chances of mechanical damage (e.g. scratching) due to roller transport

- Non-transportation, due to the film being too thick to pass through the rollers

- Sticking of films in the crossover assembly due to the soft gelatine adhering to dry crossover rollers

- Sticking of the film in the fixer and/or wash racks.

Various hardening agents are in common use, for example certain aldehydes and sulphates. However, all modern emulsions are pre-hardened as part of the manufacturing process and this greatly assists in the protection of the film in high temperature roller transportation.

Wetting agent

This is added to stimulate uniform development by reducing the surface tension between the developing solution and the film emulsion. It allows easy penetration of the developer into the emulsion, which would otherwise prove difficult (in the short period spent in the developer tank in automatic processing), due to the presence of hardener.

Some developer formulations may not contain this agent, as emulsions do contain a proportion of wetting agent added during manufacture. Most agents are detergent-based derivatives and because of this another additive is needed to combat problems that may arise due to the agent's basic property of foaming (see Antifrothant, below).

Anti-frothant

The automatic processor relies, for replenishment and recirculation, on the use of pumps. These pumps deliver developer under some pressure to the main tank. This pressured delivery together with the action of the rollers provides a very important feature of the automatic processor, that of constant agitation. However, it also raises the problem of foaming and frothing, mainly due to the presence of the wetting agent.

Therefore an anti-foaming agent is included to reduce foaming, which, if allowed to occur, would contaminate the inside of the processor.

Fungicide

The developer tank of the automatic processor provides ideal conditions for the growth and multiplication of certain strains of fungi. It provides a continuous and uniformly warm and moist area within which is a good deal of suitable food in the form of gelatine which is stripped off the surface of the film during transportation through the rollers. This removal of the emulsion is unfortunate but is taken into account in film and processor design.

Fungus growth can also take place within the various lines transporting fluids in the processor (especially in the wash tank and pipes), causing blockage and incorrect flow. It usually has the appearance of a slightly opaque, strand-like slime.

The addition of fungicide usually controls this growth, but in extreme cases it may persist. This necessitates the complete drainage and cleaning of tanks and lines with a powerful fungicide to remove the growth and any spores that may be present.

The advent of the first generation of cold water processors exacerbated this situation, as the low water throughput (about 1.5 l/min, compared to about 14 l/min in tempered water processors) caused great problems; many processors had to be converted back to mixed water machines. Second generation (so-called total cold water processors) solved this problem by recirculating the water at higher pressures but still using only about 1.5 l/min from the main supply.

STARTER SOLUTION

As stated previously, this is added to developer replenisher to produce machine tank developer, when starting the processor from 'dry'. It has two main functions:

- It depresses the pH of the developer, thus reducing the activity of the solution

- It adds bromine ions to the solution, thereby restraining the action of the developing agents on the unexposed AgBr grains (i.e. increases selectivity).

The amount to add is critical, as under- or over-addition greatly affects the developer's characteristics and therefore affects final image quality. It is usually supplied in a separate bottle, with instructions to add so many millilitres per mixed litre of developer replenisher in the machine tank.

Agents

Usually potassium bromide plus acetic acid.

COMMERCIAL PREPARATIONS

Developer chemical available from manufacturers is normally supplied as a liquid concentrate to make up so many mixed litres, and sometimes packed containing three parts, A, B and C. Each of the three parts comprises various items of the final developer that, for chemical reasons, need to be kept apart until working developer is required. It is not possible to be specific about the constituents of each part – exact formulations are normally trade secrets. However, generalisations can be made to illustrate actual solutions. Table 6.5 is an indication of the contents of developer solutions, if packed as three separate parts.

Never bring part B into direct contact with water; always dilute the solution with part A. This is important, as phenidone is insoluble in water and is kept in solution by the fact that it is mixed with monopropylene glycol. Direct mixing with water that does not contain part A will cause the phenidone to precipitate out. Unfortunately this process is irreversible.

MIXING

Developer should be mixed carefully, with due regard to the fact that both parts A and B can cause burns and part C is an irritant. Suitable protective clothing should be worn in the form of

Table 6.5 Developer constituents in commercial preparations

Part	Danger	Content
A	Causes burns	Developing agent (hydroquinone)
		Preservative (sulphite)
		Buffer + accelerator (alkali – hydroxide)
B	Causes burns	Developing agent (phenidone)
		Solvent for phenidone (diethylene glycol)
		Restrainer (acetic acid + benzotriazole)
		Restrainer (potassium bromide)
C	Irritant	Hardener (glutaraldehyde)
		Acetic acid

NB It is possible to purchase developer which does not contain glutaraldehyde and also where diethylene glycol has been replaced with monopropylene glycol which better comply with the COSHH Regulations.

gloves, aprons, etc. This is particularly relevant not only for reasons of personal safety, but also because of the Health and Safety at Work Act.

Before mixing the replenisher, check the volume remaining in the replenisher tank and ensure that there is sufficient space to accept the additional solution. Then:

1. Add the volume of water stated in the instructions
2. Slowly add the whole of parts A, B and C, in order, stirring continuously
3. Continue stirring for at least 2 minutes to give a uniform mixture.

Stirring is very important, as it prevents the formation of insoluble precipitates. It is also a wise precaution to use separate stirring rods for developer and fixer, as even small amounts of contamination may be detrimental.

Automatic chemical mixers

The use of automatic chemical mixers is advisable in order to minimise the handling of chemicals by the operator. The chemicals are supplied in bottles with foil tops. First, the cap is removed and the bottle is up-ended onto the mixer. The foil top is then pierced, allowing the chemicals to enter the machine. A measured quantity of water at the correct temperature is mixed with the chemicals, the force of the water being such that it ensures the even distribution of the chemical throughout the solution.

The advantages of automatic chemical mixers are:

- Reduction in chemical handling
- Even mixing
- Correct temperature of the chemicals
- Reduction in splashing and, as the chemicals are mixed in a closed unit,
- A reduction in chemical fumes.

It is important that anyone using this type of machinery is trained in the correct use of the particular equipment being used.

LOW TEMPERATURE CHEMISTRY

The normal range of temperatures within which developers operate can conveniently be divided into two sections. These are so-called high and low temperature, and their ranges are only relevant when considering radiographic processing (Table 6.6).

The advent of the demand for low temperature chemistry posed many problems for the designers of chemical systems, as it was still necessary to retain the same total processing cycles (i.e. 90 seconds, 2 minutes, etc.) which meant

Table 6.6 Temperature ranges

Division	Temperature	Normal pH
High temp. chemistry	31°C–39°C	9.6*
Low temp. chemistry	26°C–33°C	10.00*

* Actual values depend on manufacturer.

staying with short developing times and also retaining the same image quality.

The main problem was that of processing the film at lower temperatures for the same time, but still producing the same maximum density, contrast, speed and base + fog levels. In order to achieve this, three principal alterations have been made in the production of low temperature chemistry. These are:

1. Higher concentration of hydroquinone
2. Different restrainer
3. Higher concentration of preservative.

The increase in the hydroquinone level provides the higher activity needed at lower temperatures to give the required densities. Unfortunately hydroquinone is more susceptible to aerial oxidation and therefore requires a higher concentration of preservative. The higher pH, caused again by the large amount of hydroquinone, also has an adverse effect on the usual restrainers, requiring a change in this agent as well.

The advantages of low temperature chemistry are the much lower running costs and the fact that it is energy saving.

Practical tests

These are the subject of Chapter 10 (Quality assurance), but can be summarised as:

- pH of the machine tank developer

- pH of the replenisher tank developer (these can be plotted on a graph and any variations studied)

- Measure replenishment rates

- Specific gravity of the machine and replenisher solutions

- Sensitometric evaluation, i.e. full sensitometry; fog, speed and contrast index, visual comparisons.

SUMMARY

- For a chemical to be useful as a developer, it must possess two main properties: *conversion* and *selectivity*. It must be able to convert exposed silver bromide to metallic silver while leaving unexposed silver bromide relatively unchanged (Fig. 6.8).

- The *amplification gain* of the silver + developer system is of the order of 10^9.

- Developers for automatic processing have special features that distinguish them from their manual counterparts, and although it is possible to use auto-process developers in a manual situation, it is usually not possible to do the reverse. The *developer and the replenisher have different properties and pH values*, e.g. pH developer 10.00, pH replenisher 10.30. But they are related by the fact that:

  Developer replenisher + starter = machine tank developer

- *Developer replenisher* is used to maintain constant solution activity and quantity. There are many factors affecting the degree of replenishment required.

- *Starter solution* must be added to replenisher when initially filling the main developer tank. This is because it has two important effects. First, it increases the bromine ion concentration; second, it depresses the pH to the correct value, enabling immediate use of the processor to give correct film quality.

- A typical *developer* comprises many *agents*. Table 6.7 shows the general names of these agents, their probable chemical composition and their functions.

- Commercial developer preparations may be supplied in three parts. These can be hazardous if handled incorrectly and must be kept apart for complex chemical reasons (see Table 6.5). Ideally an *automatic chemical mixer* should be used.

Table 6.7 Developer constituents: probable composition and function

General name	Chemical used	Function
1. Developing agents	Phenidone plus hydroquinone	Selective conversion, AgBr (exposed) to metallic silver
		Also possesses the feature of superadditivity
2. Preservative	Potassium metabisulphite	Reduces aerial oxidation to a minimum
3. Accelerator	Sodium or potassium hydroxide	Gives the developer its pH value, therefore ensuring correct activity
4. Restrainer (anti-foggant)	Organic: benzotriazole	Improves developer selectivity, therefore reduces fog level
	Inorganic: potassium bromide	Also found in starter solution
5. Buffer	Boric acid + sodium hydroxide	Maintains pH within defined limits and therefore activity of developer constant
6. Sequestering agent	EDTA sodium salt	Softens hard water
7. Solvent	Water	Acts as solvent for all chemicals and by-products of developer action
8. Other additions		
Hardening agent	Reduces emulsion swelling and softening	
Wetting agent	Reduces surface tension	
Anti-frothant	Prevents foaming due to reduced surface tension	
Fungicide	Reduces growth of fungi	

If chemicals are mixed manually they should be mixed carefully, with suitable precautions, according to the manufacturer's instructions, and always with continuous stirring.

- *'Low' temperature chemistry* differs from 'high' temperature chemistry in that it has a higher hydroquinone concentration, a different restrainer and a higher preservative concentration.

- *Practical tests* listed above, are also the subject of Chapter 10 (Quality assurance).

- The constituents of developer can easily be remembered by using the mnemonic *SOAPRADS*:

    S — Solvent
    O — Other additions
    A — Alkali buffer
    P — Preservative
    R — Restrainer
    A — Accelerator
    D — Developing agents
    S — Sequestering agent.

FIXERS

The fixer bath is, in most cases, the least understood solution used in processing. It is not generally appreciated that while it is possible to produce an adequate image in a development time of, say, 10 seconds, it is not possible to completely fix the image in such a short period without the use of expensive and perhaps potentially hazardous solutions, both of which features are undesirable in a hospital setting.

In the early days of automatic processing, most of the problems associated with the chemical side of the processor were eventually traced to the fixer, so much so that the modern processor is designed primarily around the fixer solution. This in no way decreases the importance of the developer or the other processing systems, but indicates the importance attached to ensuring that the film is correctly fixed.

Previously it was stated that very rapid fixation was not possible using conventional agents; however, these agents can be used to provide, in certain situations, a 'quick look' facility. In these cases, the film must be returned for completion of the process if any degree of archival permanence is to be achieved.

For a chemical to be a fixer it must possess two properties: conversion and selectivity.
Conversion. It must be able to:

Convert unexposed, undeveloped silver halide into a form that can be removed from the emulsion layer by the water present in the fixing bath, thus rendering the image permanent.

The agent present must therefore be a silver halide solvent that produces salts that are soluble in water. This can be briefly described by the following equation:

Silver halide + fixing agent → water-soluble silver complexes + inert by-products

Selectivity. In this sense, 'selectivity' means that the agent:

Must have no effect on either the metallic silver in the developed image or the gelatine in which it is suspended.

Again, however, as with developer, it is a far from perfect world, and unfortunately all fixing agents are to some extent mild silver solvents. Only two agents are in common use:

- Ammonium thiosulphate $(NH_4)_2S_2O_3$
- Sodium thiosulphate $Na_2S_2O_3$.

Only one of these – ammonium thiosulphate – is used in radiographic processing. Other fixing agents found in use in other fields, but not in medical X-ray departments, are the alkali cyanates and thiocyanates. Even though they are very much more rapid in action, unfortunately they may have a detrimental effect on the silver image and gelatine.

The conversion process occurs in three stages when a thiosulphate is used, the middle step producing the only salt in the photographic process that is not soluble in water. This apparent disadvantage provides a useful test of whether the film is correctly fixed (this is discussed further in the next section).

Fixing solutions

All automatic processing fixers used in imaging departments are of the *ammonium thiosulphate acid hardening type*. This is significant because ammonium thiosulphate is the most rapid, easily prepared and easy to use fixing agent in terms of mixing and safety (although it still needs to be prepared and used with some care). The acid present in these fixers negates the need for a rinse or stop bath process between development and fixation and also allows the use of very efficient hardening agents which are essential when rapid drying at high temperatures is required (as in an automatic processor).

These factors mean that maintenance of the fixer pH value within fine limits is essential, and to this end all commercially available fixers have a pH range of approximately 4.2–4.9, depending on the manufacturer, and a tolerance of ±0.2 pH (approximately) about the recommended value.

Constituents

The constituents of fixer replenisher and machine fixer are listed below. Unlike developer, there is no difference between replenisher and machine tank fixer in terms of the actual agents employed, or in terms of their pH value:

1. Fixing agent
2. Acid
3. Buffer
4. Preservative
5. Hardener
6. Solvent.

Need for replenishment

As the fixing process progresses, there is a decrease in the level of the active ingredients of the fixer solution and also an increase in the level of by-products. The *fixing agent* is used up as it converts the silver bromide into soluble silver complexes, which leads to an increase in the silver concentration of the fixer. If this is allowed to climb above 7–8 g/l it results in insufficient fixation because the rate of diffusion of the soluble silver complexes out of the film falls below a minimum safe level. This cannot be compensated for by increasing the fixing time, as in automatic processing this cannot be changed.

Similarly, the *pH* of the fixer will alter due to carry-over of alkali developer in the emulsion of the film, and although the squeegee rollers of the automatic processor reduce this to a minimum, it cannot be completely eliminated. An increase in the pH value of the solution away from its ideal eventually affects the hardener, which becomes less efficient, resulting in problems with transportation of the film through the rollers as well as scratching and inadequate drying.

In the absence of corrective measures being taken, these problems would necessitate constant changing of the fixer solution to maintain consistent results, the change being necessary approximately twice as often, in a given solution, as with developer in a similar situation.

To obviate this, a certain amount of replenisher is added to the machine tank every time a film is fed into the processor. When added in the correct proportions this ensures that the level of the active ingredients is maintained at the correct concentration by adding fresh solution. It also results in removal, usually to a silver recovery unit, of the same amount of used fixer. This keeps the volume constant and also, if correctly replenished, the silver level constant (usually 5–7 g/l); this final fact ensures that the soluble silver complexes are completely removed from the film, providing pH and fixing time remain constant. It also ensures that the physical amount of fixer used is not excessive (see Ch. 10, Quality assurance). The factors affecting fixer replenishment are as follows:

- Area of film processed
- Average density of the film, i.e. amount of unexposed, undeveloped silver bromide to be removed
- Thickness of emulsion and silver coating weight
- Single or duplitised emulsion
- Type of fixing agent (in theory only, as the agent is always ammonium thiosulphate)
- Silver level required
- pH level required.

Many of the factors listed above are closely related to each other and are decided by the manufacturer in the film and chemical manufacturing process (e.g. type of fixing agent, thickness of the emulsion, silver coating weight, etc.).

Replenishment in a normal situation is usually governed by an average rate per length of film processed, and for fixer this is approximately 80–100 ml for every 35 cm. A useful rule-of-thumb guide is that fixer replenishment should be twice that of developer in any given situation, but again this depends on other factors and really an objective evaluation is the most desirable course to take. Again, as with developer, the average rate for the 35 cm length of film means that large films actually receive under-replenishment whereas small films receive over-replenishment, the net effect over a typical working day resulting in, on average, correct replenishment. A microprocessor can be programmed to scan film via a series of detectors, and to replenish correctly according to all the pertinent variables.

Fixing agent

There is only one agent used in automatic processing fixers. This is *ammonium thiosulphate*. Ammonium thiosulphate is used exclusively because of its ability fully to fix the image in a considerably reduced time compared to its sodium thiosulphate counterpart. The decrease in time is entirely due to quicker diffusion of the ammonium thiosulphate into the emulsion layers and associated more rapid removal of by-products.

Traditionally, fixing times have been quoted as multiples of a factor known as clearing time.

Clearing time

The clearing time is defined as the time taken for the 'milky' appearance of a film that is receiving fixation to just disappear, leaving the expected 'transparent' image.

Clearing times and associated fixing times for the two common agents are as follows:

Ammonium thiosulphate
Fixing time = 1.3 × clearing time
Clearing time = 8–10 seconds (approximately)

Sodium thiosulphate
Fixing time = 2 × clearing time
Clearing time = 4–5 minutes.

All the above figures are quoted for the same film type at temperatures typically found in automatic processing. Again, this indicates the superiority of ammonium-based products in terms of speed of action. Finally, one other advantage is the fact that ammonium thiosulphate fixers are always provided in liquid concentrate form. This enables easy storage and preparation of working solutions.

Sodium thiosulphate fixers, as stated previously, are not generally in use in imaging departments of the developed countries. However, it is incorrect to think that these fixers are totally unused, as in many circumstances where speed of action is not important their use is still widespread. They are also extensively used in developing countries, where they are sold in powder form.

Function of the fixing agent

The function of the fixing agent is to:

Convert unexposed, undeveloped silver bromide into water soluble silver complexes that can be removed from the film by the solvent present in the fixing bath.

When correctly carried out, this renders the image permanent, as it removes any remaining silver bromide that would otherwise begin to break down under the action of light and cause the image to fog. It also produces the 'transparent' appearance of the film, as the areas of the film that have received no exposure, if viewed directly after development, have an opalescent 'green' appearance. This is the undeveloped silver bromide that must be removed if the image is to become stable and useful on storage.

The removal of the unwanted silver bromide has several stages, described below:

Initial stage (Fig. 6.12). The film transported from the developer into the fixer still contains alkali developer within the emulsion layers. Most of the surface developer has been removed by the action of the squeegee rollers as it passes out of the developer tank (see Automatic processing, Ch.7). However, the remainder must be neutralised as quickly as possible before the fixing agent can get to work. This is achieved by the acid in the fixing bath working in the 'neutralisation zone' (Fig. 6.12).

Stage one (Fig. 6.12). When the film has passed through the neutralisation zone, the fixing agent plus other active ingredients (e.g. the hardener) diffuse into the emulsion. The rate of diffusion depends on:

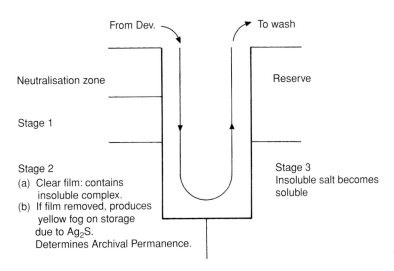

Fig. 6.12 The stages of the fixation process.

- The type of fixing agent
- The steepness of the diffusion gradient
- The temperature of the solution.

It is the temperature that determines, primarily, the speed at which fixing occurs. Once within the emulsion, the ammonium thiosulphate reacts with the silver bromide to produce silver sulphate and certain by-products.

Stage two (Fig. 6.12). The silver sulphate is further acted on by more ammonium thiosulphate to produce a simple salt of silver ammonium thiosulphate. This salt is insoluble in water. When all of the silver sulphate has been converted into this intermediate salt, the image will appear clear but is still not fully fixed. The time taken for the silver sulphate (green in appearance) to be converted into the simple salt (which is clear in appearance) is called the *clearing time*.

Stage three (Fig. 6.12). The third stage is the conversion of the simple salt, by the further action of ammonium thiosulphate, into a complex salt of *silver ammonium dithiosulphate* which is soluble in water and is washed out of the film. When all of this complex salt has been removed from the film it is considered to be fully fixed.

Reserve capacity (Fig. 6.12)

Fixation is a complex process involving many chemical reactions. As time is both limited and constant in automatic processing, it is prudent to have available a reserve capacity to ensure that correct fixation occurs. This allows for variations in, for example, temperature and replenishment that may result in prolongation of one or more of the stages just described.

If all of the intermediate salt (i.e. the silver ammonium thiosulphate) is not converted into its soluble version, fixation remains incomplete and degradation of the image will occur on storage, even though the film may have been adequately washed (poor washing being the most important factor in image deterioration on storage).

Acid

As the film is transported from the developer section of the processor to the fixer it passes through a pair of squeegee rollers that remove surplus developer from the surface of the film. However, the developer remaining within the emulsion still continues to develop the image. If allowed to continue this would lead to degraded image quality. This is prevented by:

> **The acid component neutralising the alkali developer, thus stopping development as soon as the film enters the fixing tank.**

The process is carried out in the neutralisation zone (Fig. 6.12).

An additional advantage is that the hardeners used in fixers are very pH dependent and need an acid environment in order to work at their most efficient.

Dichroic fog is a problem quoted in association with the fixing solution. It is caused, mainly in manual processing, by the continuation of development in the presence of the fixing agent and appears pink when viewed by transmitted light and green/silvery when viewed by reflected light. Dichroic fog does not occur in practice in automatic processors, as the pH value of the fixer would have to rise to such a level (certainly greater than 5.0) that the hardening action would be impaired to the extent that the film would not be transported through the processor (see Hardeners, p. 119, and Buffers, below).

Agent

The agent chosen to provide the acid content depends on which hardener is to be used. In radiographic fixers these are normally:

- Acetic acid, with aluminium chloride as hardener
- Sulphuric acid, with aluminium sulphate as hardener.

The association of a particular acid with a particular hardener should not be taken as definitive, as it is quite possible to have an acetic acid fixer with an aluminium sulphate hardener or a sulphuric acid fixer with an aluminium chloride hardener.

The choice of an acid paired with a certain hardener is made to ensure that sufficient active ions are available to produce a stable solution over a range of both storage and usage conditions.

Function

From the previous discussion it can be deduced that the main functions of the acid are to stop development by neutralising the alkali developer, and to provide the correct pH level for the hardening agent.

Buffers

As previously stated, even though the processor is designed to keep the carry-over of developer into fixer to a minimum, it cannot completely prevent it. The continual addition of even small amounts of alkali would eventually result in an increase in the pH value away from its desired level, eventually leading to problems with the hardening activities of the fixer and, if allowed to progress, would result in reduced hardening, non-drying and eventually non-transportation of the film through the processor. The classic definition of a *buffer* is:

A solution whose acidity or alkalinity is practically unchanged by dilution and which resists a change in pH on the addition of acid or alkali.

In the case of fixer, this solution is a mixture of two different agents, both of which have significant properties apart from their combined action as a buffer.

Agent

In nearly all cases, this is a mixture of *acetic acid* and one of a number of sulphite-based compounds such as *sodium sulphite* or *potassium sulphite*, to name but two. These sulphites also possess the property of exerting a preserving action on the thiosulphate complex of the fixing agent (see Preservatives, below). To this end, a fixer buffer can be considered as:

Fixer buffer = acetic acid + preservative.

Acetic acid is nearly always the acid of choice, even when sulphuric acid is used for the acid component in aluminium sulphate-hardened fix-

ers, as it has a very large buffer capacity. When acetic acid is used for the main acid content it can also act as part of the buffer combination.

Function

The single purpose of the buffer agent is to maintain the pH of the fixing solution within fine tolerances. This ensures correct neutralisation of developer contained within the emulsion as it enters the fixing tank (Fig. 6.12), and correct hardening of the emulsion by maintaining the pH level for optimum hardening action (see Hardeners, p. 119).

Preservatives

The many advantages of maintaining fixing solutions at a constant acid pH value have been established in the previous sections. Unfortunately, there is one disadvantage that cannot be conveniently ignored. If ammonium thiosulphate is placed in even a mild acid solution, it has a tendency to break down to form sulphur particles: this is known as sulphurisation. If allowed to progress, it would eventually render the fixer useless, producing a colloidal suspension of sulphur with a yellow/green 'particulate' appearance.

When the fixer is at the correct pH value, the production of sulphur particles is prevented by the preservative's active ions combining with any sulphur that may have formed to produce a soluble complex that leads to the sulphur being redissolved. This effectively cancels out any effect that the sulphur would have had on the fixing bath.

Maintenance of correct pH values is very important, as the level can have serious effects on the preservative's action:

- If the pH is allowed to rise above 5.0, a white crystalline deposit forms. This is a *precipitate of sodium aluminate*, formed as a result of the action of the preservative and the hardener. Unfortunately, it is almost totally insoluble and is very difficult to remove. In practice it is probably true to say that the problems associated with decreased hardening action would be noticed before any white precipitate is formed (Fig. 6.13).

- If the pH is allowed to fall below approximately 4.0, massive *sulphurisation* occurs due to the increased acidity. In practice the reduction of the pH to below 4.0 should not occur, providing certain simple precautions are taken during the mixing of fixer replenisher.

Normally, fixer hardener is added last to the combination of fixing agents and water. The hardener solution has a very low pH value (i.e. high acidity) of approximately 1.0–1.5. If it is added without sufficient agitation it may cause localised depression of the pH to below 4.0, resulting in the production of sulphur. This can easily be seen during the mixing process. If precipitation does occur it can, apparently, be dispersed by further vigorous agitation. This does not cause the sulphur to redissolve; it simply mixes it throughout the replenisher tank and, when left to stand (say, overnight), it precipitates to the bottom of the tank where it can be seen as a light yellow crystalline deposit (Fig. 6.13).

Again, vigorous agitation will disperse this deposit, but it will reappear when the solution is left to stand. The quantity of this deposit poses no particular problem unless it is present in excessive amounts, when it may cause partial filter blockage within the automatic processor or replenisher tank, resulting in reduced flow rate.

It is very important to reduce to a minimum aerial oxidation of the developer (see Developer preservative, p. 104). However, it is often erroneously stated that fixers do not suffer from oxidation caused by the air. The fact is that while the *fixing agent* (i.e. ammonium thiosulphate) is not affected by the oxygen in the air, the *preservative* is significantly affected, its efficiency decreasing according to the length of time of exposure. This decreasing efficiency is due to the sulphite ions combining with the oxygen to produce a sulphate which has no preserving action (Fig. 6.14).

Reduction of the sulphite preservative level in this way renders the fixing agent more susceptible to sulphurisation, even at correct pH values, due to the decrease in the available sulphite causing a reduction in the efficiency of the conversion of any free sulphur into soluble inert (as far as the fixer is concerned) complexes.

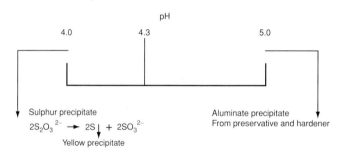

Fig. 6.13 The effect of pH on the preservative.

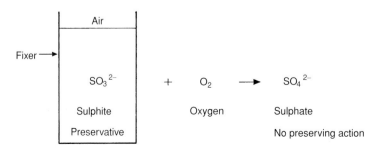

Fig. 6.14 The effects of oxygen on the fixer preservative.

In order to combat this problem:

- If possible, fit the fixer replenisher tank with a *floating lid* similar to that in use in the developer replenisher tank; this reduces the surface area of the fixer in contact with the air. To be fair, this is only required when fixer use is very low, e.g. a theatre processor.

- When preparing a solution for use in an area of very low film throughput, i.e. where there is very low fixer usage, do not make up more solution than is necessary to do the amount of work required.

In the majority of situations, auto-oxidation of the sulphite does not present any particular problem due to the high usage of fixer found in most departmental automatic processors. However, it is not unusual to find the yellow precipitate (even if only a small amount) associated with sulphurisation due to poor mixing.

Agent

In all cases this is one of a number of sulphite-based compounds, the important criterion being the number of free sulphite ions liberated when the agent is in solution. It is the sulphite ion that has the preserving action on the ammonium thiosulphate. As there are a number of suitable agents, just two will be quoted as examples: sodium sulphite (Na_2SO_3) and potassium sulphite (K_2SO_3).

Function

The function of the preservative is to prevent or reduce to a minimum the breakdown of the fixing agent into sulphur particles. This breakdown is due to the action of the acid components of the fixing solution on the thiosulphate complex, and is called sulphurisation. Any free sulphur particles produced within the solution are converted by the sulphite ions present into a soluble complex that can be reabsorbed.

Hardeners

One of the major problems associated with rapid film processing is the necessity of using high processing temperatures and high pH values to reduce processing times. This has undesirable effects on the emulsion, causing excessive absorption of the processing solution; this leads to swelling and softening of the gelatine, leaving the film in a very delicate condition. In order that the film may be processed in a roller-type processor, the emulsion must be hardened to control the moisture absorption and, therefore, swelling and softening. If the film was not hardened, even a human hair on the surface of the emulsion would cause significant scratching. Hardening is so important that it is carried out during all the following stages:

- Film manufacture
- Development
- Fixing.

Film manufacture

The film is hardened at this stage to enable it to resist the abrasions caused by packing, unpacking, loading/unloading into the cassette, etc. It would be impractical to attempt completely to protect the film from the effects of careless handling. There is sufficient hardening to afford reasonable protection, but the film is still able to absorb the developer quickly enough to develop the image in about 22 seconds in a 90-second processor.

Development

Here the film is further hardened, as part of the development process, to resist the swelling and softening caused by the high temperatures and pH values of the developing solutions. However, it is important not to over-harden at this stage, as this would make fixation more difficult by slowing down the rate of absorption of fixing solution into the emulsion.

Fixing

The hardening is continued as part of the fixing process, where it prepares the film for the wash tank. It is here that the film is brought to its final degree of hardness, so that it does not absorb too

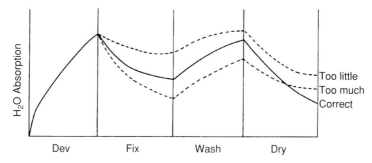

Fig. 6.15   The effects of hardening on emulsion water absorption.

much water during the washing process. If too much is absorbed the film would not become completely dry in the limited time available in the automatic processor dryer. Therefore, the amount or degree of hardening of the film in the fixer determines how efficiently the film will dry. Other factors are also significant, for example temperature, humidity, etc., but still one of the most common causes of the film coming out of the processor wet or damp is inadequate hardening, usually due either to failure to add sufficient hardening solution or to under-replenishment of the fixer.

Over-addition of the hardener can also cause problems of:

- Inadequate washing, due to reduction in the rate at which the wash water diffuses into and out of the emulsion, and consequently inadequate drying

- The archival permanence of the image. The film may be just dry enough to be handled, but may still contain thiosulphate complexes that have not been removed by washing. These decompose on storage and cause image staining to such a degree as to render the film useless.

The fixing bath is the only place where, in practice, the concentration of the hardener can be affected to any significant extent. This is due to the fact that during emulsion coating it is controlled by the manufacturer, and because hardening variations in development are not normally associated with immediate processing problems. For some reason it is all too common to discover that either no hardener or insufficient hardener has been added to the fixer replenisher. The problems associated with this occur quickly,

starting with damp films and leading eventually to the film sticking in the processor, usually just at the entrance to the dryer where the wet sticky emulsion meets the hot dryer rollers.

Figure 6.15 shows the approximate moisture absorption caused by the addition of too much and too little hardener to the fixer replenisher.

Hardener and pH values

In the section on acid it was stated that one of its functions was to provide the correct pH value for the hardener to work. The efficiency of the hardening action is very pH dependent, even small variations giving considerable changes in emulsion moisture absorption. Most conventional aluminium-based agents have their maximum characteristic hardening between a pH of 4.3 and one of 4.6, with a peak at 4.4 (Fig. 6.16). Consistent pH values above and below these limits soon manifest themselves as damp films coming out of the processor and, while it is difficult to produce low pH values (unless due to very poor mixing), high values (i.e. above 4.6) are easily produced by under-replenishment (Fig. 6.16).

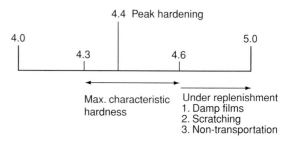

Fig. 6.16   The effect of pH on the hardening characteristics of fixer.

Agent

The agent used as hardener varies according to which manufacturer produces the fixer. It is paired with a particular acid. This pairing increases the stability of the particular hardening agent in use. There are two principal aluminium-based compounds to be found in fixing solutions:

- Aluminium chloride ($AlCl_3$) with acetic acid
- Aluminium sulphate ($Al_2(SO_4)_3$) with sulphuric acid.

The active ingredient of the combination is the aluminium ion.

Function

The function of the hardening agent is to control the swelling and softening of the emulsion (i.e. moisture uptake), thereby allowing roller processing, high processing temperatures and rapid drying times. It also protects the film from moderate forms of mechanical damage that may occur during processing.

The control of moisture uptake is achieved by the aluminium ions causing cross-linking of the gelatine polymer within the emulsion, thus keeping the chain-like molecule 'tightly packed', even though its spiral structure tends to unwind when placed in water.

Solvent

Again, as with developer, this is almost always water. Normal tap water is more than adequate but the use of a filtered supply from the output side of the water mixing panel has the added advantage of reducing to a minimum the presence of particles of grit, dirt, etc., that may scratch the emulsion if allowed into the machine tank of the processor.

Tap water has all the advantages and disadvantages stated in the section on developers earlier in the chapter, but in this case there is the additional problem associated with the presence, in the film emulsion, of the only non-water soluble salt in the photographic process.

COMMERCIAL PREPARATIONS

Fixer replenisher available from manufacturers is normally supplied as a liquid concentrate to make up so many mixed litres, typically containing two parts. These parts are either marked 'A' and 'B' or 'Replenisher' and 'Hardener' (part A corresponding to the replenisher and part B to the hardener). Unlike developer, some manufacturers provide replenisher and hardener as separate items and require a separate order for each (rather than combining them in one complete pack). The exact contents of each part are normally trade secrets, but in general are as summarised in Table 6.8.

It is very important never to add concentrate part B (i.e. hardener) to concentrate part A (i.e. replenisher), as an instant precipitate of aluminium forms, 'plates' onto any metallic components and is extremely difficult to remove. This precipitate can form even when there are relatively low concentrations of part A, so it is good practice to add only hardener to correctly diluted part A (see below, Mixing).

MIXING

Ideally, automatic chemical mixers should be used. Fixer should be mixed carefully with due regard to the fact that both parts can cause burns. Suitable protective clothing should be worn in the form of gloves, apron, glasses, etc. These basic precautions are often ignored, and while it is considered tedious by some people to put on protective aprons, etc., it does prevent fixer

Table 6.8 Fixer contents in commercial preparations		
Part	Danger	Content
A Replenisher	Causes burns	Fixing agent Acid
		Buffer
		Preservative
		Solvent
B Hardener	Causes burns pH 1.0–1.5	Hardener Acid

splashes burning holes in clothing and prevents dermatitis from splashes on the skin.

Before mixing the replenisher, check the volume remaining in the tank and ensure that there is sufficient space to accept the additional solution. Then, to manually mix:

- Add the volume of water stated in the instructions.

- Add slowly the whole of part A (or the part marked 'replenisher') with continuous stirring.

- Add the whole of part B or, if the hardener is supplied separately, the correct amount according to the instructions. This is usually so much hardener per mixed litre of solution; typical volumes are 25 ml per litre. Thorough stirring at this stage is vital to prevent localised production of insoluble sulphur particles.

- Continue stirring for at least 2 minutes to ensure a uniform solution mixture.

Some manufacturers offer the option of diluting the replenisher either 3 : 1 (i.e. three parts water to one part fixer) or 4 : 1, the choice depending on the particular application the fixer will be used for. This also alters the amount of hardener required. There is no advantage in under-diluting fixer in an attempt to obtain more rapid fixing; in fact the amount of water present is vital as this is the solvent for the final product of the fixation process. An easy proof of this is trying to fix a film in a dish of concentrated fixer; no matter how long the film is left it will not clear. However, if this concentrate is slowly diluted with increasing amounts of water, the film will clear rapidly.

Temperature ranges

The temperature of the fixer is vital if correct fixation is to be assured. Simply: the higher the temperature the shorter the fixing time. Within certain limits, there is an almost linear relationship between increasing temperature and decreasing fixing times. In most cases it is not possible to alter fixing times during automatic processing, therefore accurate temperature is essential.

Fixer temperatures are closely related to developer temperatures, and in an ideal situation the temperature of both solutions should be identical (e.g. 32°C). However, in practice it is quite common to find slight variations between the two; in general, the maximum variation allowable is that the fixer should not be more than 2°C lower in temperature than the developer.

All commercially available solutions are designed to work in the range 26–39°C, allowing alterations in fixing times away from the approximate 22 seconds found in 90-second automatic processing. This means that these are suitable for use with both high and low temperature developer chemistry. Problems may occur at the lower end of this temperature range, but these probably would not be visible until after a period of storage. Increasing to a 2-minute processing cycle may prove to be the cure for this situation if this is convenient from a departmental point of view.

Practical tests

These are the subject of Chapter 10 (Quality Assurance) but can be summarised as:

- pH of the machine tank fixer
- pH of the fixer replenisher
- Measure replenishment rates
- Measure silver concentration levels
- Specific gravity of the machine and replenisher solutions
- Sensitometric evaluation.

SUMMARY

- For a chemical to be a fixer it must possess two main properties, *conversion* and *selectivity*. It must be able to convert unexposed, undeveloped silver halide into a form that can be washed from the emulsion, but it must not degrade the newly developed image or affect the gelatine in which it is suspended.

- All fixers used in automatic processors are of the *acid hardening* type, using ammonium thiosulphate as the fixing agent. This agent produces the most rapid fixers without having to resort to the cyanates (although these have a more rapid action).

- The *pH* of the fixer must be maintained within fine limits to ensure rapid neutralisation of the alkali developer and to provide the correct environment for the hardener to work.

  Automatic processor fixer has a pH range of 4.2–4.9, and should be maintained within 0.2 of its recommended value.

- Fixer *replenisher* is important as it is used to maintain solution activity and quantity. There are many factors affecting the degree of replenishment required and these are listed in the main text.

- A typical fixer comprises many agents. Table 6.9 shows the general names of these *agents*, their probable chemical composition and their function.

- Commercially available fixer may come in two parts, marked 'A' and 'B' or 'Replenisher' and 'Hardener', respectively. These concentrates should never be mixed without the *correct amount of water* being added first.

- When mixing chemicals, follow carefully the manufacturer's instructions, wear *protective clothing* and use continuous stirring.

- Fixer *temperature* is closely related to developer temperature and should be no more than 2°C cooler than the developer.

- *Practical tests*, given as a list above, are the subject of Chapter 10, Quality assurance.

WASHING

The washing process is important, since production of the final image can be severely damaged by neglecting the simple process of adequately washing the film. In automatic processing it is not usually possible to significantly alter wash rates, other than to forget to turn on the water supply to the processor; and in any case the water flow to the processor is normally set by the engineer on installation, according to the manufacturer's recommendations. It must also be remembered that the water supply can be responsible for assisting in the control of other important processor functions, for example developer temperature control, etc. (see Automatic processing, p. 132); therefore altering water flow to increase the efficiency of the wash process may affect other systems whose immediate importance outweighs the necessity for better washing.

In general, however, when operating correctly, the processor is designed to more than adequately wash the films for conventional purposes.

Function

The function of the washing process is to remove from the film emulsion fixer that has not been used in the conversion of unexposed, undeveloped silver bromide into soluble complexes, and also to remove the remainder of the soluble silver

Table 6.9 Fixer constituents: probable composition and function		
General name	Chemical used	Function
Fixing agent	Ammonium thiosulphate	Conversion of undeveloped AgBr into soluble silver complexes
Acid	Acetic or sulphuric acid	Stops development
		Provides correct pH for hardener
Buffer	Acetic acid + preservative	Maintains pH of solution
Preservative	Sodium or potassium sulphite	Reduces sulphurisation to a minimum
Hardener	Aluminium chloride + acetic acid Aluminium sulphate + sulphuric acid	Controls emulsion water absorption
Solvent	Water	Acts as solvent for fixer chemicals and by-products of fixation

complex salts that have not been removed by the water present in the fixing solution.

The removal of these substances is of vital importance, as it is the level of these salts in the film after washing that determines its archival permanence.

ARCHIVAL PERMANENCE

Archival permanence is defined as:

> **The length of time a film will store without significant deterioration in its image quality.**

In practice, the tests carried out in most imaging departments are quite inaccurate and only give a vague idea of safe storage times. The normal bands considered are: less than 5 years; 10–20 years; 20–25 years and more than 25 years. These bands are then measured using a colour comparison chart. More accurate methods of determining archival permanence are available but require some knowledge of chemistry and access to chemical analysis equipment (e.g. BS 1153/1955). It is traditional to test for residual thiosulphate to measure archival permanence, as this proves to be most convenient. (See also Chapter 10, Quality assurance.)

The salts responsible for image degradation are silver complex salts and residual thiosulphates.

Silver complex salts

These consist of the intermediate insoluble silver salts that remain in the emulsion due to inadequate fixing (i.e. not all have been converted to the soluble silver complex salt for some reason), and the soluble silver complex salt that has not yet been dissolved by water. Washing the film is not going to remove the insoluble salt, as this is a problem of poor fixing, but it will remove the soluble complex. This soluble complex deteriorates with time to form a silver sulphide which produces an overall yellow/brown 'fog', therefore its reduction to a low level is important.

Residual thiosulphate

This is the remaining ammonium thiosulphate that is present in the emulsion. If not completely removed it decomposes to produce a very mild acid which attacks the silver image and converts it to a silver sulphide. This results in a yellow/brown staining and image fade, due to the reduction in the amount of silver forming the image.

It is traditional to test for archival permanence by estimating or actually measuring the amount of residual thiosulphate present in the emulsion after it has been dried. This test is chosen because ammonium thiosulphate is present in the largest quantities, it is easier to detect by chemical test, and both the soluble silver complexes and the thiosulphate are removed from the emulsion at the same rate.

STAGES OF WASHING

Washing is essentially a diffusion process that occurs in the following three stages:

- Due to the concentration gradient that exists between the high salt concentrations within the emulsion as compared to the water in the wash tank, the residual salts diffuse out of the emulsion.

- The dissolved salts within the water around the film are removed by the constant circulation of water within the automatic processor wash tank.

- The contaminated water within the wash tank is replaced by fresh incoming water, thus helping to maintain the high concentration gradient required to wash the films to the correct degree.

Diffusion of the salts out of the emulsion occurs until an equilibrium situation exists between the concentration in the emulsion and the concentration in the wash water around the film. In theory, the decrease in the thiosulphate content of the film follows an exponential curve with the result that no matter how long the film is washed there is never a zero thiosulphate count. However, this is of no practical significance as the lowest thiosulphate count possible depends on the proportion of other dissolved salts in the wash water. To carry this argument further, it seems logical to use demineralised water to wash the film to its ultimate extent but, if this is done, excessive swelling of the gelatine occurs; this destroys the capillaries within the emulsion and causes sludging in the wash tank.

In practice even the most efficient washing systems do not approach the level of the emulsion salt content equalling that of the water supply. This is mainly due to the short washing times found in automatic processors and the fact that there is no need to wash to such high standards. Most modern processors will comfortably wash to 175 mg of thiosulphate per square metre, which, in average storage conditions, gives more than 25 years' archival permanence.

Factors affecting wash rate

Most of the factors affecting a film's wash rate are beyond practical control, as they are a function either of processor design or of the chemical composition of the water supply. However, for the sake of completeness, the following list gives the most significant factors (and a brief explanation where necessary):

- *Steepness of the concentration gradient*
  This is the difference in the concentration between the salts within the emulsion and those in the wash water. The steeper the gradient, the more rapid the washing.

- *Rate of water flow*
  The more rapid the water change, the more rapid the washing, as this keeps the concentration gradient high and provides agitation.

- *Degree of agitation*
  High agitation levels provide high levels of fresh water to the surface of the film, helping the factors above.

- *Temperature*
  In theory, an increase in water temperature provides quicker washing. However, in practice there is little choice that can be made, as

wash temperature is a function of individual processor systems.

- *Degree of hardening*
  This is a function of fixation, and in a correctly operating processor is constant at a pre-determined level. Over-hardening of the emulsion results in poor washing, due to salts in the emulsion having difficulty in diffusing out. Under-hardening results in over-absorption of water, giving transportation problems.

- *Time in the wash tank*
  This is of little practical significance, as it is constant in an automatic processor and depends on the time cycle as a whole.

- *pH of the wash water*
  This is of no practical significance.

Many of these points are interrelated and dependent on factors such as processor design, chemical design, and the degree of archival permanence required from the stored image.

Films are conventionally kept for 8 years after the conclusion of treatment, with the following three exceptions:

1. Obstetric records are kept for 25 years

2. Records of those with mental illness are kept for 20 years

3. Children's films are kept for 8 years after the last entry, or until the child reaches 25 years of age, whichever is the longer.

Microfilm archiving systems are designed to provide this level of permanence but still require careful monitoring of residual thiosulphate contents.

SUMMARY

As this is only a short section, a lengthy summary is unnecessary; however, the following points are significant:

- The wash process is carried out to *remove* soluble *silver complex salts* and residual *fixing agent* from the film emulsion.

- The degree to which a film is washed, in most cases, determines its *archival permanence*.

- There are both objective and subjective *tests* to determine archival permanence, the most common one in imaging departments being the residual thiosulphate test.

- Washing is a continuous three-stage *diffusion process*, the rate of which depends on a number of closely related factors.

- The testing for residual thiosulphate is especially significant for *microfilm archival systems*.

SILVER CONSERVATION

Silver conservation has always been desirable. It has assumed significance in recent years due to the increased financial constraints placed on the imaging department and the widely varying price of silver. It has been estimated that the photographic industry consumes about 40% of the total silver used, and that approximately 66% of this is recoverable. The main reasons for carrying out silver recovery are as follows:

- Silver is a diminishing natural resource that requires conservation

- Effluent that contains high silver concentrations can cause ecological damage and may contravene local water regulations

- The high price of silver can sometimes bring profitable returns.

METHODS OF SILVER RECOVERY

A number of methods of silver recovery are available. For the sake of completeness the main methods are listed below; some are easier to utilise than others and the choice of method will depend on local circumstances, amount of fixer used, financial return expected, staff available, etc.

- Collection of used fixer
- Metal (ion) exchange
- Electrolytic recovery
- Recovery directly from the fixer
- Precipitation
- Collection of old films.

Collection of used fixer

This is perhaps the easiest and most straightforward of the methods listed. A number of specialist companies will collect the used fixer in containers and the silver is recovered and refined elsewhere. Credit can be given either for an estimated silver concentration at the time of collection, or for the assayed quantity after refining. Most reputable collectors will provide an estimate on collection and an assayed valuation as a check of the true silver content. This has the advantage that silver recovery takes place in a controlled fashion. It must be remembered that under the Environmental Protection Act (1990), the onus is on the person arranging the collection to ensure that a reputable firm is used and that the company is licensed to dispose of the used fixer.

Metal exchange

When a silver salt solution is brought into contact with a base metal (i.e. steel wool, zinc, etc.) the base metal is replaced by the silver, and the base metal ions are released into solution. The sludge produced can be collected and dried, and the silver refined. In a steel wool silver recovery unit this principle can readily be exploited. A steel wool cartridge of 5 kg can, theoretically, recover 20 kg of silver; in practice, an amount between 5 and 15 kg should easily be obtained. Figure 6.17 is a simplified diagram of such a unit.

The steel wool is held in a plastic container and the processor fixer overflow is connected directly to the unit via a bypass valve. This prevents the overflow of fixer should the unit become blocked. As the fixer passes over the steel wool in the cartridge, metal exchange takes place and the silver is deposited as a sludge. A secure lid is essential to prevent the escape of fumes. The unit should be kept in a well-ventilated place away from the general working environment.

To ensure maximum efficiency, particular attention should be paid to the following points:

- Ensure that the steel wool remains below the fixer solution level. This reduces oxidation of

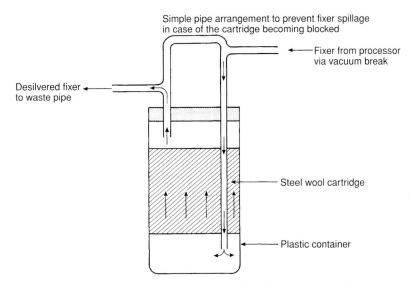

Fig. 6.17 Diagrammatic cross-section of metal (ion) exchange in the silver recovery unit.

the wool and ensures that any build-up of heat caused by that oxidation is kept to a minimum.

- Ensure that solution flow through the cartridge is at the correct speed. Too high a flow will reduce the efficiency of recovery.

- Monitor the outflow for the presence of residual silver. This can be done by a computerised monitoring and metering system which automatically tracks the flow of silver through the system. Silver estimating papers can be used for a manual check on the effluent but these can be unreliable.

- The fitting of a similar unit in tandem may improve the efficiency of the whole system.

- Remove exhausted cartridges as soon as possible.

Although this method is cheap and easy to run, some significant problems exist, such as the danger of clogging the cartridge and discharging iron ions into the drains. Modern systems overcome this problem by mixing all chemical waste and jetting the solution down the drain under pressure, to prevent sludge build-up. The variable workload experienced in most departments could mean that the automatic processor, working under peak load, would flood the cartridge, and silver would go to waste.

Theoretical efficiency is of the order of 95%, but in practice 70% is a more realistic target.

Electrolytic recovery

Providing the unit is working correctly, very pure silver is produced by this method (of the order of 95–98% purity) very little further refining is required and there is the possibility of re-using the fixer. It is based on the principle that when two electrodes (usually a carbon anode and a stainless steel cathode) are placed in a used fixer solution and a direct current is passed between them, positively charged silver ions (Ag^+) are attracted to the cathode, where their charge is neutralised and they plate out as metallic silver (Ag). If the current is increased, the silver is deposited faster. However, if the current is too high or the silver concentration too low, the ions cannot get to the cathode fast enough and 'sulphiding' occurs. This is a black layer of silver sulphide which can eventually stop the plating process altogether. These factors influence the construction of the two types of electrolytic units.

Low current density

Originally these units were left in situ in the fixer tank of manual processing units. They use large electrodes with a very low current in order to reduce the risk of sulphiding. However, the current must not be too low, as no transfer of the silver ions will occur at very low current densities. Units are available for use in conjunction with automatic processors which have a small throughput of films and therefore would make high current density units uneconomic.

High current density

In high current density units the fixer solution is under constant agitation. This allows operation at a higher current and the use of a smaller surface area cathode without the same danger of sulphiding. Agitation is achieved by rotation of the cathode and/or the anode, a separate stirring device or by bubbling air through the solution. This has the advantage of bringing fresh silver ions close to the surface of the cathode and speeding up the rate of deposition of metallic silver.

The output of these units can range from 5 to 40 g per hour.

It is possible to use more than one silver recovery unit in such a way that the effluent from the first unit passes into the second for further recovery, which is particularly useful in busy departments. It is also possible to connect several processors to a single silver recovery machine.

Regular checking of the silver levels and adjustment of the current density is required to avoid sulphiding and thus ensure maximum silver returns. However, in most departments this would be too time-consuming and units are set to a current value that corresponds to an 'average' silver concentration of the fixer.

Modern units have solved this problem by incorporating a microprocessor that monitors silver concentration and adjusts the current supplied to give maximum returns. In addition they can indicate the amount of silver which has been recovered and when the cathode (which can be disposable) requires changing.

Recovery directly from the fixer

The recovery unit is plumbed directly into the processor fixer tanks. As fixer is circulated

through the unit, silver is recovered using the electrolytic method. This maintains very low levels of silver in the fixer solution and therefore reduces the amount of silver that passes into the wash water. The unit can have an additional metal exchange unit attached to the outlet to ensure that the discharge from the recovery unit remains below the legal minimum.

Collection of old films

It should not be forgotten that old films have a considerable amount of silver content. A number of specialist companies operate collection services for quantities of used film. The company will normally offer a price for each kilogram of film to be collected; this will depend on an estimate of the recoverable silver available and whether the films are in envelopes or not. Credit is normally given against the assayed value of the recovered silver, minus an amount for the service provided by the company.

ESTIMATION OF SILVER YIELD

This is fraught with many problems and no firm indication can be given, as numerous variables are involved: for example, the average density of the films after processing, the average silver content of the fixer before recovery, the average silver content of the fixer after recovery, the silver content of all the different types of emulsion being used in the department, the exact efficiency of the recovery methods in use, etc., etc.

It has been suggested that there are, on average, approximately 4 g of recoverable silver per square metre of film used. While this may be a reasonable guide, it does not take into account advances in emulsion technology resulting in lower silver coating weights or local variations in the factors mentioned above. It seems reasonable to suggest that an estimate for the potential amount of recoverable silver is made over, say, a 6-month period and that this is compared to actual returns.

The amount recoverable can be estimated by multiplying the amount of fixer used in the period by the average silver content of that fixer, less an amount for fixer that has been wasted. Of course this is only very approximate but may serve as a rough guide. It has also been suggested that the fixer leaving the recovery unit should be regularly monitored: providing that this is somewhat below 1 g/l, this is an acceptable indication of an adequate standard of recovery.

Chapter 7

Automatic processing

INTRODUCTION

The final step in the production of the X-ray image is processing, either manual or automatic. This final procedure is as vital as any other link in the imaging chain. No matter how good the radiographer, the film or the screens, the final result is made or marred in processing.

The purpose of this chapter is to look at the advantages of automatic processing. The inside of an automatic processor is usually a mystery to those who use it: to elucidate this mystery a processor is constructed from scratch. Recent developments of automatic processors are also considered.

Modern automatic processing produces few film faults and these are almost always the same. These faults are listed, as are general film faults.

MANUAL PROCESSING VERSUS AUTOMATIC PROCESSING

Before automatic processing is discussed, it is worthwhile to look closely at manual processing and then to examine the reasons why automatic processing was an inevitable and valuable progression.

Time

Table 7.1 illustrates the relative differences in time required by manual and automatic processing. The times given are average values.

Convenience

In manual processing there are nine distinct steps:

1. Unloading the film
2. Loading the film onto a hanger
3. Development
4. Stop bath or rinsing
5. Fixing
6. Washing
7. Immersion in a wetting agent
8. Drying
9. Reloading the cassette, possibly with wet hands.

These nine steps provide nine opportunities for damage to the film or screens to occur.

In automatic processing, the list comes down to the following three:

1. Unloading the film
2. Inserting into processor
3. Reloading the cassette.

Table 7.1 Time requirements of manual and automatic processors		
Process	Manual	Automatic
Development	3–5 min	22 s
Stop bath or rinse	10–20 s	Nil
Fixing	10 min	22 s
Wash	15 min	22 s
Drying	20 min	24 s
Total	(approx.) 50 min	90 s

In daylight handling systems the list is as follows:

1. Inserting the cassette into the system.

Thus, in a centralised daylight system, one single operation is all that is required!

Economics

Very often, justification has to be made for the purchase of an item such as an automatic processor. Listed below are the various considerations of manual versus automatic processing:

- Automatic processing eliminates all hangers and their replacements.

- There is little or no difference in the electrical consumption of the two systems, assuming there is thermostatic control on the manual system and there is an electrical dryer. Indeed, with modern processors the current drain could be typically 6 A.

- Water consumption is significantly lower in automatic processors than in manual processors. Water in a manual system has to run continuously in the wash tank. Typically, this can be about 12–15 l/min. With modern energy-saving devices, automatic processors use about 1.5 l/min, and that only while there is film in the processor.

- Film wastage can be reduced simply because of standardising the development process.

- Chemical costs for both manual and automatic systems will be approximately the same, as long as correct replenishment procedures are applied.

- An average darkroom technician can process about 5 m^2/h manually. With an automatic processor this increases to 15 m^2/h.

- There is a considerable saving in space using automatic processing.

As a very rough guide, if film consumption of the department reaches 10 m^2 a day (about 138 24×30 films), then automatic processing is the cheaper of the two systems, bearing all the above in mind. The saving can be as much as two-thirds of the cost of manual processing.

Advantages of automatic processing

All the factors which can influence the photographic quality of the radiographs are kept within very fine limits. Automatic processing therefore provides consistent, uniform results:

- Time in the developer, fixer, wash and dryer is constant, due to a controlled drive system.

- In normal conditions the temperature of all the solutions is unaffected by outside conditions.

- The quality and the quantity of the solutions are maintained to a high standard, due to automatic replenishment.

- Pump-driven circulation of the processing solutions along with continuous movement of the rollers ensures constant agitation, giving uniform penetration of the chemicals into the emulsion layer of the film.

- Constant dryer temperatures, along with even distribution of the drying air, ensure even drying and a uniform surface quality of the film.

- Because of all these factors, coupled with the exposure latitude of modern X-ray film, satisfactory results can be obtained with exposure discrepancies as great as ± 25%.

- Very short exposure times are to a large extent made possible by absolute uniformity of these factors, which is almost impossible to achieve with manual processing.

In short, the modern automatic processor may be considered as its own compact environmental control unit.

THE AUTOMATIC PROCESSOR

Evolution of the automatic processor is still continuing, albeit with help of the ubiquitous computer. There are now many and various types of processors, all with idiosyncrasies that would be impossible to describe. It would seem best to start with a description of a typical automatic processor and look at some ways, in mechanical and engineering terms, that the sometimes complex problems have been tackled. It should be stressed that no processor exactly like the one described here exists. Students should familiarise themselves with the automatic processor in their own department. Ample literature exists which describes particular makes and types of processors.

A TYPICAL AUTOMATIC PROCESSOR

A typical automatic processor consists of a number of separate but interrelated systems. These can be listed as follows:

- Film entry system
- Transport system
- Chemical and recirculation system
- Replenishment system
- Water system
- Dryer system
- Electrical system.

Each of these will considered in turn and a processor will be 'constructed' using the equipment suggested.

Film entry system

Every processor must have some apparatus which will take the film into the processor. Usually this is linked to the replenishment system so that the act of feeding the film into the processor activates the replenishment pumps for a period of time. An ideal film entry system would consist of:

- A pair of rollers
- A microswitch, above the rollers.

These would be combined to make a system as illustrated in Figure 7.1.

There are many versions of the microswitch: examples include an infrared light beam which is stopped by entry of the film; a trip wire, which in turn operates a microswitch; even a steady

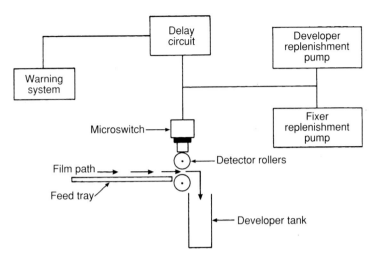

Fig. 7.1 Film entry system.

stream of air, which again is interrupted by the film's entry.

In this 'ideal' processor, the lower roller is fixed and the top roller, which is of significant weight, has a small movement allowed. When a film leaves the feed tray, the top roller is forced upwards. If the microswitch has been set correctly this movement will trip the switch and activate a number of electrical systems.

Subsystems

The feed system is usually interrelated to:

- The replenishment system
- Some warning system.

In basic automatic processors, the action of inserting the film activates a relay which switches on the replenisher pumps. It becomes obvious that if a simple switch is used the processor is only capable of recognising the *length* of the film being inserted. The pumps are therefore only working when the film is going through the film entry system.

The warning system is used in many different ways, but it is usually used to tell when the next film is to be inserted (i.e. when the first film is clear of the entry rollers). This warning could be a bell, a buzzer, a warning light or a safelight over the feed tray which is switched off as the film goes into the processor.

Transport system

In automatic processors the transport system consists of a series of rollers which are used to move the film through the processing tanks (see Fig. 7.2). This system also relies on an electric motor driving all the racks at a constant speed. The constant speed is very important, so the drive system will be a common one to ensure that there is no possibility that, for example, the developer rack will move faster than the fixer rack.

The rollers can be arranged in many and varied formations, but essentially they will be arranged in either deep tanks or shallow tanks.

There are advantages and disadvantages to both of these systems, but the major one relates to cost. A shallow tank system will be simpler

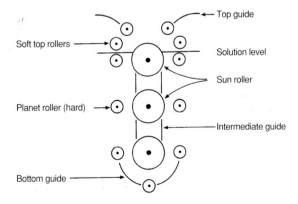

Fig. 7.2 Rack arrangement.

and cheaper to make and run, as far fewer rollers are used. Usually the capacity (i.e. the number of films per hour) is lower than a deep rack system.

The deep rack system can be of very high capacity, but will usually be more costly because of the large numbers of rollers involved.

In term of processing quality there is little to choose between the two systems.

Within the racks will be found guide plates. These plates are used to keep the film within the transport path. They are made of stainless steel or plastic and have to be kept meticulously clean, particularly if they are above solution level. If lengthwise scratches occur on the film, it is almost 100% certain that guide plates are the cause.

Rollers fall into various types. They can usually be described as hard or soft.

Hard rollers

These can be made of stainless steel or (nowadays more usually) paper wound on a stainless steel core and impregnated with an epoxy resin. This explains why great care must be taken when cleaning this type of roller. Coarse cleaning materials can seriously damage the surface of the 'paper' rollers, causing permanent damage. This will cause marks to be printed on films.

Soft rollers

These are usually found in crossovers in the machines. They can be used as 'squeegees' to squeeze the excess chemicals off the films and thereby reduce carry-over of chemicals. They are usually constructed of a neoprene-type substance (not rubber, which is not inert as far as processing chemicals are concerned).

Chemical system

This system comprises the tanks for developer and fixer and the allied subsystems.

The tanks themselves must be constructed of some inert material such as stainless steel or plastic. They act as containers for the developer, fixer and wash water.

Once developer and fixer have been made up in the processor and the processor started, the chemicals have to be circulated constantly and maintained at the correct temperature.

It can be seen from Figure 7.3 that the chemical system is closely interrelated to the other systems, i.e. the replenishment, water and heating systems. In any processor, no matter what type or make, this interrelationship must exist.

Circulation of developer

In the recirculation system, the developer is constantly passed through the following (see Fig. 7.3):

- Thermostat
- Temperature gauge
- Heat exchanger (water system)
- Circulation pump
- Heater
- Filter.

Thermostat

Note that *thermostat* and *thermometer* are not synonyms. The thermostat *controls* the temperature; the thermometer merely *measures* the temperature.

The thermostat is the device which senses the temperature of the solutions. Once the operating temperature is set, the thermostat will automatically switch the developer (or fixer, if

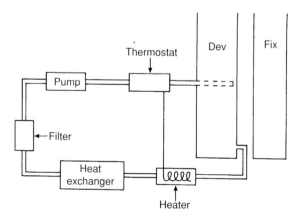

Fig. 7.3 Recirculation of developer.

fitted) heater off and on at the appropriate temperature.

Thermometer

It is extremely important to have a constant display of developer temperature wherever possible. In some machines, the thermometer may be replaced by a simple light which will constantly cycle between off and on, indicating that the correct set temperature is being maintained.

Heat exchanger

This is also part of the water system. The developer and water circulate separately through this device. The operation of the heat exchanger is fully described under the water system (p. 138).

Circulation pump

This pump forces circulation of the developer through the various devices listed above. Note that ideally the developer would be taken from the bottom of the tank, circulated through the system, and then be brought back to the middle of the tank. It can then be forced through a 'spreader' which will ensure adequate spread of the solution throughout the tank.

Heater

The developer is passed over this small, relatively low consumption in-line heater. The heater, in turn, is linked to the thermostat.

Filter

It is certainly not obligatory, but the use of an in-line filter helps to keep the developer cleaner. The filter could be as simple as a stainless steel or plastic mesh, or as complex as a sophisticated renewable device filtering down to about 25 μ.

Developer recycling

It is possible to recycle developer and although at present this may not justify the cost of the necessary equipment, if disposal legislation changes then it may become more viable.

Advantages of recycling

- Reduces developer consumption by 70%
- The filtering of the developer can help to reduce the replenishment rate
- Reduces the amount of waste produced.

Disadvantages of recycling

- Additives or specially formulated developers may be required

- Chemical 'lid', made up of an immiscible fluid, which is required to reduce aerial oxidation.

Fixer circulation system

The fixer circulation system is constructed in almost exactly the same way as the developer. If the processor is a so-called 'cold water' processor there will certainly be an in-line heater and thermostat. If it is a 'tempered water' processor (i.e. it uses both hot and cold water), a heat exchanger would certainly be used in the fixer circulation system to utilise waste heat from the developer, via the water system, to maintain the fixer temperature (Fig. 7.4).

A filter is sometimes found in a fixer circulation system.

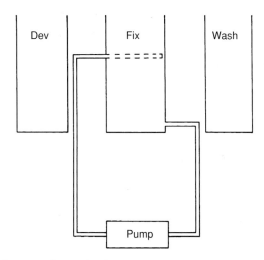

Fig. 7.4 Fixer recirculation.

Replenishment system

The replenishment system preserves both the *quality* and *quantity* of the chemicals in the processor. The basic system consists of:

- Replenisher tanks
- Filters
- Replenishment pumps (linked to the film entry system; see Fig. 7.5).

Replenishment tanks

These must be constructed of an inert material such as stainless steel or plastic. While the developer and fixer tanks perform exactly the same function (i.e. they hold the replenisher), they differ in their construction.

The developer tank has a floating lid on top of the developer replenisher. This is used to reduce the auto-oxidation of developer replenisher solution. Remembering that developer is a reducing agent and has an affinity for oxygen, care must be taken to reduce auto-oxidation at every opportunity.

It is a sensible practice to make up only enough developer replenisher to last for about a fortnight. It is also necessary to keep the floating lid clean and not to allow any oxidation products to build up on the surface.

In addition to the floating lid, there is usually a cover. The cover is there to prevent easy access for dust or dirt.

The fixer tank will exactly duplicate the developer tank, apart from the floating lid.

Filters

Filters are usually found in the line from the tanks to the processor. These can be a simple stainless steel mesh, to catch large particles which may block the pump or the line to the processor.

Replenisher pumps

These pumps are operated from the microswitch in the film entry system. The pump can be a single electric motor which drives two impellers, forcing the solutions up to tank level. There is always a device either in the pump itself or in the replenisher line which allows individual adjustment of the developer and fixer replenishment rates.

It is very important that there should be no flow back into the replenisher tanks from the main processor tanks. This can be prevented in two ways, either by creating a break in the line so that the replenisher is fed over the top of the tank via a 'hook', or by having a one-way valve in each line.

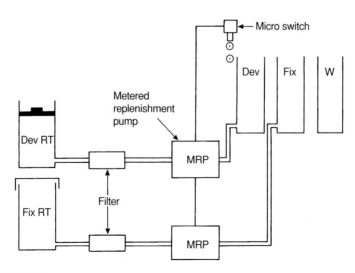

Fig. 7.5   Replenishment system.

In shallow tank processors a simple feed system can be used. This consists of a bottle containing the replenisher, inverted over the processing solution. When the level of the solution drops, the solution from the bottle automatically refills the solution back to the preset level. Replenishment then stops (Fig. 7.6).

Fixer recycling

To enable the recycling to take place, the fixer is continuously circulated through an electrolytic silver recovery unit.

Advantages

- The silver content is reduced and therefore the replenishment rate may be reduced
- There is less silver transported to the wash water.

Disadvantages

- Due to the relatively low cost of fixer there is very little cost saving
- Fixer that has been through an electrolytic system may produce unpleasant fumes
- There may be a problem of blocked pipes and sulphiding.

Ecologically optimised system (EOS) technology

A recent innovation is the introduction of a second fixer tank in the processor. The tank next to the developer holds used fixer and is directly fed by the next tank which holds fixer replenisher, the film passes through both tanks. This system reduces the concentration of silver in the wash to less than 1 mg/litre, and fixer replenisher, fixer

waste and water consumption can be reduced by as much as 35%.

Water system

This is sometimes considered to be the simplest of the systems within the processor. This is certainly not the case.

The water system is influenced by the type of processor, i.e. whether it is a 'cold water' processor or a 'tempered water' system.

Tempered water processor

This will consist of the following components (Fig. 7.7):

1. Cold and hot water supply
2. Filters
3. Mixing valve
4. Flow gauge
5. Temperature gauge
6. Heat exchanger (developer)
7. Heat exchanger (fixer).

Cold and hot water supplies. Ideally, these should be of equal pressures, about 34 474 newtons per m^2 (5 psi) being the minimum pressure which is acceptable. The ideal solution would be to have two water header tanks of the same height. Unfortunately this is not always possible and pumps (to increase the pressure) or valves (to reduce the pressure) may have to be considered.

Filters. Ideally, both hot and cold water supplies should be filtered to avoid contaminants in the water and to avoid clogging the mixing valve.

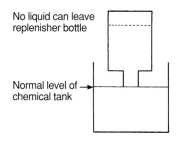
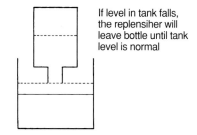

No liquid can leave replenisher bottle

Normal level of → chemical tank

If level in tank falls, the replensiher will leave bottle until tank level is normal

Fig. 7.6 Replenishment system in shallow tank processor.

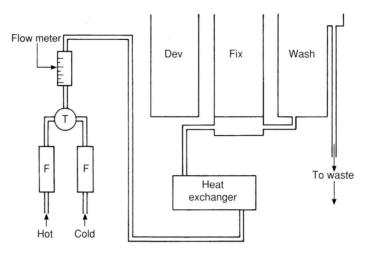

Fig. 7.7   Water system.

Mixing valve. This is a water/temperature control valve operated by a thermostatic motor. It is capable of controlling water flow and temperature to a very high degree, typically ± 0.5°C.

When the valve is set for temperature it will maintain a constant flow of water. Most valves have a cut-off device which will not allow only hot or only cold water to flow into the processor.

Flow gauge. This is a gauge utilising a stainless steel float. The scale is calibrated to indicate the flow rate of water into the processor.

Temperature gauge. Not obligatory, but certainly it is very useful to see at a glance the operating temperature of the water in the processor.

Heat exchanger. This is a box containing a series of tubes through which water and developer (or fixer) run. The tubes are totally separate (Fig. 7.8).

The purpose of the heat exchanger(s) is to absorb any waste heat from the developer and to finely control the developer temperature. If the heat exchanger is used in the fixer, the reverse operates. The waste heat from the developer is passed to the water and then re-absorbed by the fixer.

When the heater is switched on:

• The developer reaches its correct temperature.

• The thermostat recognises that the correct temperature has been achieved (for example 36°C) but there is a considerable amount of residual heat left in the heater and this will continue to (over) heat the developer.

• The heat exchanger comes into play to maintain the wash water at least 3°C below the developer temperature.

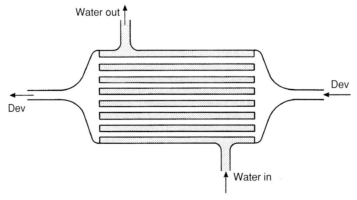

Fig. 7.8   Heat exchanger.

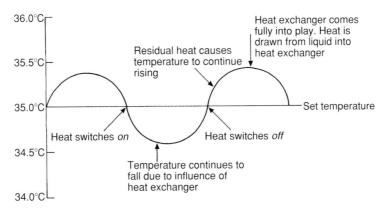

Fig. 7.9 Graph of thermostat response.

- The excess heat from the developer is now absorbed by the cold water in the heat exchanger and the overswing in developer temperature is brought down.

- When the developer temperature reaches the correct temperature the thermostat recognises this and switches the heater on.

- However, there is a slight delay in heating, and the developer temperature goes below the correct temperature until the heater takes full effect.

If a graph is drawn of this response it will be seen as a sinusoidal curve, keeping the swing of temperature under very fine control (Fig. 7.9).

Dryer system (Fig. 7.10)

This is almost a totally self-contained unit. It comprises the following elements:

- Roller transport system
- Blower
- Heater
- Thermostat
- Filter
- 'Air knives'.

Roller transport system

This is driven from the main drive shaft to ensure that the speed of the film through the dryer is the same throughout the processor.

Blower

This unit generates the air flow used in drying the film.

Heater

The blown air is driven over the heater.

Thermostat

The thermostat is used to set the temperature of the drying air. This is usually about 50°C. It should be noted that there is also a safety thermostat incorporated in the dryer. This cannot be

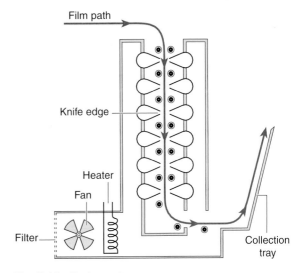

Fig. 7.10 Drying system.

adjusted, and it will switch the dryer heater off if the temperature exceeds 60°C in order to prevent damage to the film emulsion.

Filters

On some processors, the air coming into the blower is filtered as well as the outgoing air to the heater.

Filters are fairly essential in the dryer area, as any dirt blown into the air system will be directed onto the film surface.

'Air knives'

These are used to increase the velocity of the air as it strikes the film surface.

They use the principle of the Venturi effect. This means that air at low velocity forced through a large diameter bore will increase in velocity if it is forced through a smaller diameter bore.

It should be noted that the dryer transport section is constructed such that the first third of the section is used to heat the water carried in the film and make it vaporise. The second third is used to blow the water vapour away from the film surface very rapidly. The last third is there for spare capacity.

If a film leaves the dryer wet, it is very rarely as a result of incorrect dryer temperature. It is nearly always a result of poor fixation, perhaps because of under-replenishment or lack of hardener. Film should dry, if all the parameters in the processor are correct, at fairly low temperatures.

Electrical system

The combination of water and chemicals with electricity could be fatal. Therefore great care must be taken in the installation of an automatic processor. Various standards are applied in different countries, but they all specify precautions to be taken at installation in terms of electrical safety, any pollution effects (i.e. discharge of developer and fixer) and connections to water supplies.

Standby system

There is also a requirement for processors to have a standby system to reduce running costs.

The standby system will automatically shut down some operations of the processor, as listed below, if a film has not entered the processor for a predetermined interval. In a 90-second processor, a typical interval would be 2 minutes.

Water supply

This will be reduced to an absolute minimum, typically 5 litres per minute. This will be just sufficient to maintain the correct developer temperature via the heat exchangers.

Circulation system

The developer circulation system must be left on, to maintain the correct temperature. Sometimes fixer circulation is shut down.

Transport system

The processor transport system will stop completely until the next film is inserted when an infrared detector will automatically restart the processor or the standby system is recycled.

Dryer

This again is shut off until the next film is inserted, or until the standby system has recycled.

Recycling is not always fitted to a standby system, but it is a useful addition. The system switches the machine on if a film has not entered the processor for a predetermined interval, usually about half an hour. This action prevents the drying out of the crossover rollers (which can create 'pie' lines; see p. 144), prevents the dryer and perhaps fixer getting too cold, thus ensuring that the processor is always ready for use.

Processors may run on three phase or single phase electricity supplies. It is essential that, before installation, close contact is maintained between the company representative and service engineer to ensure that the correct electrical supply is installed, along with the other installation requirements.

The final processor 'built' from the descriptions contained in the chapter is merely a composite of all the parts outlined.

Cold water processor

The description of the cold water processor is almost identical to that of the tempered water processor (above) apart from some minor details. The water system will differ in that only cold water is used. This can simplify and reduce the installation costs for the automatic processor. A mixing valve is not required. Because of this, the description is based mainly on the tempered water system.

The cold water processor (Fig. 7.11) uses in-line heaters to heat both the developer and fixer. Any waste heat from the water, developer and fixer is utilised by heat exchangers. Some processors even use waste heat from the dryer to heat the water. Therefore, the cold water processor is a large energy saving device.

Processor cycle time

Once the leading edge of a film has entered a processor the cycle time is determined by the length of time that it takes for the leading edge to appear at the other end of the processor; this is sometimes referred to as 'leading edge to leading edge time'. The cycle time is fixed by the manufacturers and the early processors had a time of 7 minutes, which was soon reduced to 3.5 minutes and later to 90 seconds or less. Variable cycle processors are now available which allow the operator to select the cycle time from a choice of several times. One manufacturer produces a machine with four variables, the fastest being 38 seconds and the slowest 3.5 minutes.

As outlined at the beginning of the chapter, no processor available on the market looks and operates exactly as the above processors. Features from many different types and makes of machines have been incorporated, to give a general description. It is up to the individual student to study the machine in his or her own department and to become familiar with it.

MICROPROCESSOR CONTROL

In an automatic processor there are many tasks which should really be regularly monitored, for example:

- All solution levels

- All solution temperatures

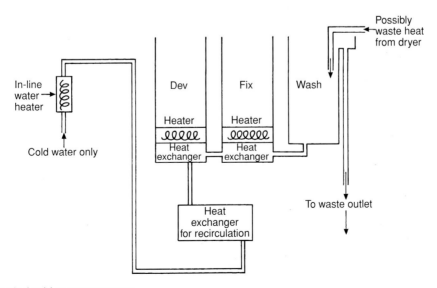

Fig. 7.11   A typical cold water processor.

- Dryer temperature

- Area of film entering the processor

- Transport speed

- Interrelationship between different speeds and replenishment (called 'intelligent replenishment').

A microprocessor is ideal for such tasks. It can monitor all of the above, the results being displayed on either a LCD or LED display. In some automatic processors the microprocessor even has the ability to communicate with an external service engineer's computer, and can run a program to check the function of the electrical system of the automatic processor.

Perhaps the most important task is the ability to monitor the *area* of the film entering the processor (Fig. 7.12). Processors used only to measure the *length* of the film entering the processor, and replenishment was set as an average figure for the department throughput. With both length and width of the film being measured, a very high accuracy of replenishment can be achieved. The measurement is usually done by a series of reed switches, microswitches or infrared light. The length of the film can easily be measured as in the normal processor; the special switches measure the width. It is then a simple calculation to determine the area.

CINE PROCESSING

The cine processor has essentially exactly the same features as a conventional processor, apart from its unique ability to transport small film in long lengths.

Cine processors are usually capable of handling:

16 mm film
35 mm film
70 mm film
75 mm film
100 mm film (roll and cut film)
105 mm film.

The processor can be totally microprocessor controlled, with a display communicating any faults to the operator. It can be used, for example, in cardiology units or for processing mass miniature chest radiographs.

DAYLIGHT SYSTEMS

The term 'daylight system' was coined in the 1970s and tends to be very misleading. Perhaps the name of these systems should be: 'A film handling system capable of loading and unloading cassettes, without recourse to darkroom facilities.' All daylight systems on the market are capable of doing just this.

Why select daylight over conventional processing?

- Better working conditions for staff
- Better use of staff time, enabling more patient contact
- Faster image production

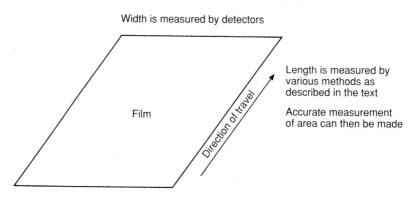

Width is measured by detectors

Film

Direction of travel

Length is measured by various methods as described in the text

Accurate measurement of area can then be made

Fig. 7.12 Determining area of film being processed.

- Less opportunity for damage to cassettes or films
- Fewer cassettes required due to the faster loading/unloading times.

The systems

Different daylight systems have different design philosophies, but they all have one important factor in common. Without exception, they all use cassettes which are dedicated to that system. These cassettes are not interchangeable between different makes of daylight system.

Some makes are suitable for use easily as a manual cassette, but will transfer immediately for use in the daylight system. This gives the user the benefit of being able to purchase (and use) cassettes prior to the purchase of the actual daylight system.

Some makes have to use film which is in a dedicated package, to fit a particular daylight system. These packs can be loaded into the daylight system in actinic light. The films are notched to accommodate the mechanical requirements of the daylight system. Others use conventional NIF film, which must be loaded into a magazine in a darkroom prior to the magazine being inserted into the daylight system.

Daylight systems are split into two different types: dispersed systems and centralised systems.

Dispersed systems

The dispersed daylight system is in two parts:

1. A series of loaders, of different sizes, which contain the film to be loaded into the cassettes
2. The unloader for the cassette, which is mounted on top of the processor.

The loaders can be distributed around the imaging department, in different areas, allowing easy access for the radiographers. The cassettes are then returned to a central processor (with unloader) for processing.

Centralised systems

The centralised system contains the film magazines, the loading and the unloading mechanisms, all directly linked to the automatic processor.

In this case the radiographers return the cassette to the daylight system, where the cassette is unloaded, the film fed into the processor and the cassette reloaded.

In the more recent daylight systems, microprocessors have been totally incorporated. They:

- Control the routine, day-to-day running of the automatic processor in the daylight system
- Keep a record of all film used
- Monitor all service interventions
- Record the electrical/electronic and mechanical state of the machine.
- Can communicate with external computers (notably the service engineer's) to produce a record and to run self-test programmes
- Have LED or LCD displays, giving details (for example) of faults occurring, size of cassette/film being used, etc.

The film is either:

- Automatically unloaded from a cassette via a lightproof, spring-loaded slot, the springs are opened by pressure on the unloader and the film falls down and is transferred into the automatic processor

or

- A conventional cassette is used which is opened and the film is extracted by the use of suction pads and transferred to the automatic processor.

In a centralised system, the cassette is then reloaded with a correct-sized film. In the case of the decentralised system, the empty cassette is then taken to the correct-sized loader, where the film is automatically loaded into the cassette.

A comparison of the systems

Advantages and disadvantages of centralised systems

Advantages

- The system is quick to use
- Loading and unloading take place in one place

- The cassettes can be used with a conventional automatic processor

- The size of the darkroom can be reduced, thus saving space

- In small departments the unit can be sited adjacent to the imaging room, enabling the radiographer to maintain contact with the patient

- There is no requirement for a dedicated darkroom technician, resulting in a better working environment for staff.

Disadvantages

- The initial cost of the system

- If one part of the system breaks down the rest of the system cannot be used

- If not correctly sited or if the correct number of units is not purchased there may be workflow problems due to queuing at the unloaders.

Advantages and disadvantages of decentralised systems

Advantages

- More flexibility in the siting of equipment
- Film dispensers and processors can be in separate areas
- The film dispensers can be purchased in various sizes to suit the requirements of each work area
- If a unit breaks down, an alternative dispenser or film size can be used
- The size of the darkroom can be reduced to save space.

Disadvantages

- The initial cost of the system
- The staff may have to walk further to process the films
- Depending on the siting of the equipment, there may be less efficient use of staff time.

PROCESSING FAULTS

With the modern automatic processor, very few faults can be said to be typical, but most are connected with the transport system.

Longitudinal scratches

These are usually connected with the guide plates in the racks. The problem can sometimes be in determining which rack is responsible.

It is almost impossible for *transverse* scratches, occurring across the direction of travel, to be caused by an automatic processor. They are almost certainly caused in the darkroom.

Pie lines

These are marks caused by chemicals partially drying out on rollers, or even by an eccentric roller in a chemical tank.

The term 'pie line' is applied because the marks repeat at intervals equal to the diameter of the roller causing them. This provides some clue as to how to trace the fault. There are sometimes different sizes of rollers within the processor; at least the diameter of the roller can be assessed and checks made.

White or black 'spots'

Usually caused by a breakdown on the surface of a 'hard' roller, sometimes due to excessive cleaning.

These types of marks can sometimes resemble calculi or phleboliths and can lead to misleading diagnoses.

To trace the fault can be a long and time-consuming job. Each roller must be checked for surface damage.

Drying marks

These can only be viewed by reflected light. They appear as dull longitudinal lines running down the film in the direction of travel.

They are caused by dirt or dust blocking part of the air knife.

Non-drying

While not strictly a mark, non-drying can be the most troublesome fault in automatic processing.

It is almost never caused by a fault in the dryer; the fault tends to be in the fixer.

The first check to make should be a measurement of the pH and silver levels of the fixer. If these are high, then a check should be made of the replenisher pumps.

GENERAL FAULTS

Unfortunately from time to time faults occur on films which can eventually be traced to the way that the films have been handled or to the way in which they have been processed. Included below are some typical film faults and some ways in which it may be possible to decide how to cure them.

The list is equally applicable to manual and to automatic processing.

HIGH DENSITY MARKS

Black 'splashes'

These generally have the appearance of a 'splash' on the film. They can have two separate causes:

1. The film has been splashed with developer before development. The area of the splash now develops faster than the surrounding area and leaves an area of high density on the film.

2. The film has been splashed with water before development. The water softens the emulsion and allows developer to enter the area quickly, again leaving an area of high density on the film.

In both of the above cases, the marks can also be produced by liquid spills on the 'dry' bench.

Black marks

These can be of many and various shapes; because of this, only the major types have been listed.

Crescent shaped

Almost always caused by bad film handling techniques. They are usually caused by the dark-room technician gripping the film too tightly between thumb and forefinger. This presses the thumbnail into the film. This action sensitises the emulsion, as the silver halide crystal is sensitive to pressure. When the film is processed, the sensitised area will show up as a black crescent shaped mark.

Note: This mark can sometimes be *white*, if the film has been handled badly *before* exposure.

Black fingerprints

Usually caused by the darkroom technician having developer or water on his or her hands. This practice can lead to further problems if the intensifying screens are handled with wet hands, as the marks produced are not removable.

Static marks

These also can be of many and various shapes. However, if examined under a magnifying glass, the point of origin of the discharge can usually be clearly seen.

The worst example is 'tree static', where large discharges can cover large areas of the film. The discharge produces distinctive marks looking exactly like the branches of a tree.

Trying to cure static problems can be difficult and time-consuming. There are, however, some classic causes of static:

- A combination of a 'formica'-type bench and vinyl floors can lead to static problems. The cure here is to cover the bench with an oil-based linoleum.

- A very dry atmosphere in the darkroom can also produce static. The easiest way to prove that dryness is the cause is to boil a kettle in the darkroom.

- A technician wearing a man-made fabric, particularly nylon, can easily produce static.

- The insertion and extraction of film into a cassette can produce quite high electrical charges. Screen cleaner, of the appropriate make, usually has anti-static properties and therefore it is worth cleaning the screens on a regular basis using screen cleaner.

Surface marks

These marks are usually single-sided and adhere to the surface of the film. They are obvious, but the causes are many; two examples are:

1. Algae in the wash tank. The wash tank is usually static overnight and is the perfect breeding ground for algae.

    Some processors now incorporate an automatic drain for the wash tank if the processor is shut down to reduce this problem. A simple way of retarding the growth of algae is to regularly rinse the wash tank out with a solution of Domestos (mixed 0.5 of Domestos to 3 of water). Make sure to *thoroughly* rinse the tank out afterwards with clean water.

2. Bits of emulsion, etc., in the developer, fixer or wash tank.

    If the surface marks persist, the only real cure is to check each tank in turn and clean it and also check the roller surfaces.

Pressure marks

As silver halide is sensitive to pressure, marks can be produced which are at first very difficult to trace. It should be noted that these can be *white* or *black*, depending on when the original mark was produced and how much pressure was exerted.

They have no special distinguishing marks and will appear randomly over the film. They can be caused by film being stored incorrectly (i.e. horizontally instead of vertically), or simply by poor film handling.

As a general guide, white marks are caused *before* exposure, black marks are caused *after* exposure.

The only procedure to follow is to check the handling and storage routine in the darkroom.

Radiation or light fogging

Again, these marks will appear at random over the film, but they will usually cover larger areas than marks resulting from other causes. Some identifiable causes are listed below:

- If the film has been fogged through material, paper for example, a faint image of the material can usually be seen on the film.

- If a similar mark occurs on a film of the same size, check to see if the marks can be superimposed. If they can, almost certainly the film has been fogged by X-radiation while in the box.

- Black marks around the edge of the film point to light leakage in the cassette, or indicate that the film box has been opened in white light.

Overall high density

Possible causes are listed below:

- *Lead-based paint.*

- *Some varnishes.*

- *Formaldehyde.*

- *Carbon monoxide.*

- *Mercury.* Never use a mercury thermometer in the darkroom.

- *Developer.* Try to ensure, wherever possible, that films and photographic chemicals are not stored in the same room.

- *Heat.* About 20°C is the maximum temperature acceptable for three months' storage.

- *Time in storage.* Films have a limited shelf life, and fog will increase with age.

- *Faulty or incorrect safelights* can cause an overall fog. Check the wattage of the bulb (no greater than 25 W). Check the filter type to match the sensitivity of the film. Check for cracks, etc., in the filter.

- *Background radiation.* A simple check would be to leave an unexposed film, sealed in a light-tight envelope, in the suspect area for 3 weeks. If the film is fogged after processing, radiation should be suspected.

LOW DENSITY MARKS

White 'splashes'

These can have two separate causes:

1. Fixer has been splashed onto the film before

development. The area of the 'splash' is therefore cleared before the area can be developed.

2. There is grease or oil on the surface of the film. Although this may seem unlikely, if a technician eats, for example, a packet of crisps and then handles a film, oil is carried to the surface of the film. The oil acts as a barrier to the developer and a white mark is produced.

In both the above cases, the marks can be produced by liquid spills on the 'dry' bench.

White marks

These can be many and various in shape and cause; because of this, only the major types have been listed.

Crescent shaped

For details, see under High density marks, above.

White fingerprints

Usually caused by the technician having fixer or oil-based products on his/her hands. This practice can lead to further problems if the intensifying screens are handled with the fingers, as the marks produced are not removable.

Pressure marks

For details see under High density marks, above.

Sharply defined marks

These are usually associated with artefacts inside (or closely adhered to the surface of) the cassette. If any artefact is present on the screens, the light output from the screens is reduced or cut off completely. This, in turn, produces a white mark on the film. Screen marks always appear in the same position on the film, for obvious reasons, which means that the films can be superimposed with the marks in position.

It is worth stressing that developer, fixer and water can damage intensifying screens irrevocably, producing consistent but ill-defined marks on the films. Physical damage (scratches, nail varnish deposits, etc.) can also produce marks on the films.

It may be necessary to view the screens under ultraviolet light to see the marks.

OTHER FAULTS

There are various other faults which are not easy to categorise.

Dichroic fog

This appears as a pink stain if the film is viewed by transmitted light, and greenish blue when viewed by reflected light.

It is caused by development still continuing in the fixer. This will happen if the fixer pH is too high. This is usually caused by excess carry-over of developer into the fixer.

If using a manual system, check that intermediate rinsing is carried out between the developer and the fixer or, better still, that a stop bath is used in this position. Glacial acetic acid solution makes a very good stop bath. It stops development immediately and does away with intermediate rinsing.

Dichroic fog almost never occurs in an automatic processor.

Milky white stain

This is due to the film being inadequately fixed, either because the film has not been in the fixer for long enough or because the fixer is grossly under-replenished.

Brown stain

The stain usually appears after a period of storage of the processed film. It is due to inadequate washing of the film. It can sometimes be cleared by refixing the film.

In both a manual and an automatic system it is always wise to do regular archival testing (see p. 203) to check washing efficiency.

The above list is by no means comprehensive, but it should help in identifying the more common faults which occur.

REFERENCE

www.medical.agfa.com

Chapter 8
Sensitometry

CHAPTER CONTENTS

INTRODUCTION

Sensitometry as a photographic science has been credited to two Americans, Hurter and Driffield, who first proposed a form of evaluation of the performance of photographic material in the late 19th century.

Sensitometry requires that the photographic emulsion be exposed to a specified light source for specified times and then the emulsion is processed under closely controlled conditions. The resultant densities produced on the film are then measured and plotted against a logarithmic scale of the exposure. The standard illuminant is an incandescent electrical light source of a specified brightness and spectral emission.

The main application in radiography is how the film will react to X-radiation, and to the light produced by the intensifying screens.

The exposure of the photographic emulsion to controlled exposures and controlled processing conditions is a fundamental of all photographic procedures. It is imperative that the student appreciates the factors which are involved and understands simple logarithmic relationships.

HOW TO DEDUCE DENSITY

Density can be defined as:

The amount of blackening on the film.

As a statement of fact this is correct. Mathematically, however, density is a logarithmic value. It can easily be obtained by deriving two simple ratios from Figure 8.1.

No light-transmitting material is completely transparent, and therefore some light is always absorbed in its passage through the material. In Figure 8.1, the light travelling from the light source (the *incident* light, I) has been reduced in *intensity* as it passes through the X-ray film to the eye of the viewer (the *transmitted* light, T).

Opacity

$$I/T = 100/10 = 10$$

The value 10 is known as the *opacity*.

Opacity will always be greater than unity and can reach quite high values. It is, again, a term which is not used (correctly) in radiography.

It is important to realise that in the example above, simple integers are used. Opacity could be expressed to two or three significant figures. Additionally, the figure obtained from the ratio would prove difficult to illustrate graphically.

It is easier to make a graphical representation of numerical values when the numbers are expressed as logarithms.

Density

Consider the value of 10, obtained for opacity. The log value of 10 is 1.0. This log value, 1.0, is the density of a film when the opacity is 10, therefore:

Density is the log of the opacity.

There are some important relationships about density; these are shown in Figure 8.2 and are as follows:

- That the silver weight of density on the processed film is related linearly to the blackening on the film, a factor which assumes great importance if films are being sold for silver recovery. A film with high densities (e.g. an extremity film) will contain significantly larger amounts of silver per unit area than, for example, a chest film.

- There is an interrelationships between the values, and opacity is going to reach very high numbers when the value of density is 4 (i.e. opacity will be 10 000).

- Only 1% of the incident light reaches the viewer's eye at density 2. In other words, 99% of the incident light is being absorbed by the film.

In addition:

- Density always increases with exposure (with *one* exception, *solarisation*, see p. 165).

- The eye responds to tonal changes logarithmically. (This relationship can only be accidental, but it helps.)

- Density, because it is logarithmic, is very easy to manipulate mathematically. Density 1 + density 1 = density 2.

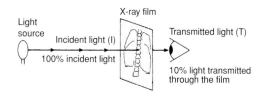

Opacity	$= \dfrac{\text{Incident light}}{\text{Transmitted light}} = \dfrac{I}{T} = \dfrac{100}{10} = 10$
Density	$= \log_{10}$ of opacity $= 1$ (i.e. the log of the reciprocal of (i.e. $\log_{10}$ of 10) transmission ratio)

Fig. 8.1 Determining density.

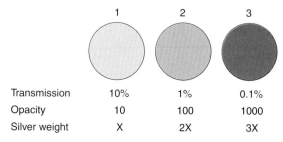

	1	2	3
Transmission	10%	1%	0.1%
Opacity	10	100	1000
Silver weight	X	2X	3X

Fig. 8.2 Density: interrelation of silver weight, opacity and transmission.

PRODUCTION OF THE CHARACTERISTIC CURVE

In the literature the characteristic curve is variously called:

- A D log E curve
- An H and D curve (after Hurter and Driffield)
- A log It curve.

All of these terms refer to the same curve.

To draw this curve, the axes are labelled as follows:

- Density is represented on the vertical (y) axis of the graph.

- The horizontal (x) axis carries the (relative or absolute) logarithmic value of the exposure, sometimes called the relative log exposure axis, or the log It (i.e. intensity multiplied by time) axis (Fig. 8.3).

Because it is a logarithmic value, each increase of log 0.30 represents a doubling of exposure, and each decrease of log 0.30 is equal to halving the exposure.

There are a number of methods of producing the characteristic curve, each with its own advantages and disadvantages. Each will be considered in turn. It is assumed that the initial curves will be produced using the simple relationship of doubling the exposure, usually for 11 steps.

Time scale sensitometry

The kV, mA and distance are kept constant and the time of the exposure is varied, always by a factor of 2. This can be done either by simply

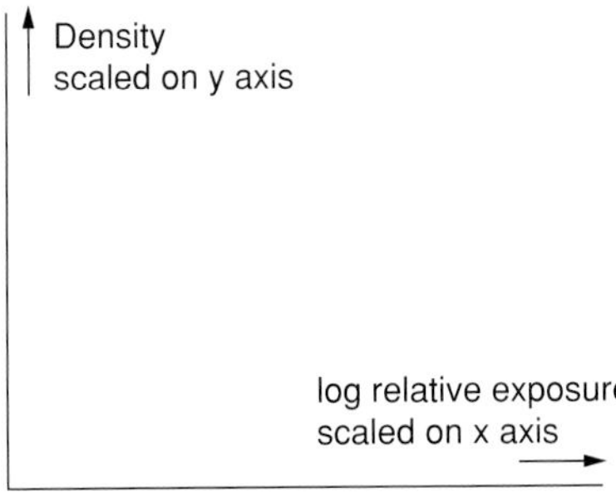

Fig. 8.3 Establishing axes for characteristic curve.

doubling the time of exposure on the X-ray set, or by covering the cassette with lead rubber and exposing it section by section. In this case the first part exposed will have received the most exposure, the last part, the least. Eleven exposures are sufficient to provide enough points on the characteristic curve to plot a reasonable graph, although 21 would be ideal (this point is considered later in the chapter).

Advantages

- It is possible to process films at a known time interval after the test and therefore prevent varying latent image problems.

- It is possible to process the film with the lower densities entering the processor first of all, thereby reducing 'bromide drag' which can cause streaking over the lower densities if the higher densities are processed first.

Disadvantages

- It has already been established that 11 exposures, doubling exposure in between exposures, will be adequate to produce the curve. If we start with 0.1 s as the first exposure we end up with the following series:

0.1, 0.2, 0.4, 0.8, 1.6, 3.2, 6.4, 12.8, 25.6, 51.2, 102.4

The experimenter has to have either a unique timer on the X-ray set, or be an extremely accurate worker with a stopwatch.

- Using this range of exposures, or even one beginning with 0.01 s, *reciprocity failure* (see p. 153) would almost certainly occur. After a time-consuming and difficult test the result could well produce a curve which, in the higher densities, does not resemble a characteristic curve at all.

- The test is time consuming to perform.

Intensity scale sensitometry

This could be carried out using the same procedure as time scale sensitometry except that the kV and distance would be constant but the mA values would be altered (i.e. constant time, varying mA).

It is more usually performed by varying the *height* of the tube in relationship to the film, using the inverse square law to perform the calculations to vary the intensity of the X-ray beam reaching the film. This technique requires great accuracy in the X-ray set, in the calculations and making of the measurements

Advantages and disadvantages are as for time scale sensitometry (above).

Calibrated step wedge

This method involves the use of an aluminium step wedge which has been calibrated in a specific way. The wedge should have a layer of copper on the base to help create a more homogeneous beam.

It is the calibration of this wedge which is most important; it also requires considerable expertise in the calculations for its construction. It has already been established that to produce a characteristic curve we have to keep to a doubling of exposures between steps.

Many people think that making a wedge with regular (i.e. 1, 2, 4, 8 cm increments) steps would give the same exposure increase, i.e. halving the exposure. Unfortunately, this relationship does not hold because of the differential absorption of the aluminium. The wedge has to be very precisely calibrated so that each step on the wedge produces an exact and regular increase or decrease in exposure. If the wedge is made with these precise calibrations, which demand very high engineering tolerances, it can be a very useful device.

Advantages

- The step wedge can be made with any number of steps and as long as accuracy has been observed in the specification and manufacture, an accurate characteristic curve will be produced.

- The step wedge can be reused.

- It can be used with different screen film combinations.

- It is possible to process films at a known time interval after the test and therefore prevent varying latent image problems.

- It is possible to process the film with the lower densities entering the processor first of all, and thus reducing 'bromide drag' which can cause streaking over the lower densities if the higher densities are processed first.

Disadvantages

- Because of the stringent specifications, a large calibrated step wedge can initially be expensive.

Sensitometer

A sensitometer is simply an exposure device which prints a pre-exposed negative directly onto the film. A sensitometer merely simulates, as nearly as possible, the spectral emission of the intensifying screens in use in the department. Sensitometers exist in many forms, from simple three patch sensitometers to large (and expensive) 21 step negatives for printing.

Whichever one is chosen, care must be taken that the light output of the sensitometer matches the spectral sensitivity of the film. It would be pointless to use a blue-emitting sensitometer with an orthochromatic (green-sensitive) film. The result produced would be invalid. The sensitometer allows the users to prepare their own step wedges easily, but it must be checked regularly to make sure that the unit is performing correctly. Figure 8.4 shows the 21 step wedge produced by a typical sensitometer.

Advantages

- Quick and easy to use.

- It can be used with different screen film combinations.

- It is possible to process films at a known time interval after the test and therefore prevent varying latent image problems.

- It is possible to process the film with the lower densities entering the processor first of all, thus reducing 'bromide drag' which can cause streaking over the lower densities if the higher densities are processed first.

Disadvantages

- The initial cost of the equipment is high.

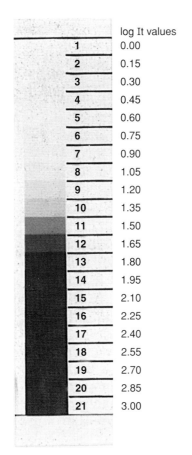

	log It values
1	0.00
2	0.15
3	0.30
4	0.45
5	0.60
6	0.75
7	0.90
8	1.05
9	1.20
10	1.35
11	1.50
12	1.65
13	1.80
14	1.95
15	2.10
16	2.25
17	2.40
18	2.55
19	2.70
20	2.85
21	3.00

Fig. 8.4 Typical sensitometer-produced 21 step wedge.

Pre-exposed step wedges

These are produced by a number of manufacturers. They are films which have been exposed by the manufacturer in a very accurate sensitometer. Films used for this type of work should have stabilised latent image storage and will be usable (after the film has been stored for a while) for a short period of time. This is why this type of film has a very short shelf life, usually of the order of 6 months.

The reason that the films are stored before release is that immediately after exposure there can be a number of ways in which the latent image can react. It can begin to fade, or remain the same, or even, over a short period, intensify. To overcome these variations, pre-exposed film is stored for a period before it is released. This factor must be taken into account when films are exposed in the department as well. It should be noted that some films cannot store a latent image for a long period of time.

Advantages

- Quick and easy to use.
- The films receive a constant, pre-determined exposure.

Disadvantages

- The cost of the films
- The films have a short shelf life.
- Can only be used to test processor consistency.

Reciprocity failure

This is sometimes referred to as the Swarzschild effect.

As long ago as 1876 two researchers, Bunsen and Roscoe, suggested that a relationship could be placed on E (effective exposure) and I (the light intensity) and t (the time of the exposure.)

They expressed the relationship as:

$$E \propto It$$

Swarzschild then modified this formula in the late 1890s to:

$$E \propto Itp$$

where p was a constant for each emulsion, but varied from one emulsion to another.

These experimenters discovered that a very long exposure to light does not produce the predicted blackening when related to a very short exposure time. The predicted reciprocity failure for a medical X-ray film would be a film which was stable at short exposure times, with an apparent loss of speed (less blackening) at very long exposure times. The only time a screen film encounters long exposure times to light is in the darkroom. Reciprocity failure at long exposures reduces the effect of long handling times in the darkroom safelight.

As Swarzschild had discovered, this effect can vary enormously between different makes of film, but all manufacturers try to ensure little or no reciprocity failure at normal exposure times in radiography. Modern theory of latent image formation can account for this effect far more readily.

It should be noted that this effect is only apparent where the exposure is due to light from the intensifying screens. With direct exposure to radiation, the X-ray quanta have such high energy, when compared to light, that they produce a latent image immediately in the silver halide grain.

Number of steps

There are three common types of grey scale (or photographic step wedge) produced. They are:

1. The three patch wedge
2. An 11 step wedge
3. A 21 step wedge (usually referred to as a root 2 wedge).

All have a role to play, but the 21 step wedge gives the best results as it gives the user a far better curve. The reason it is referred to as a root 2 wedge is that the difference between each exposure is the previous exposure multiplied by root 2, or 1.414. This fits onto the log It scale very well, as the log value of root 2 is 0.15 (see Fig. 8.5).

Calibration of a step wedge

Aluminium step wedges can be used as a test tool even though they produce totally arbitrary density steps. This step wedge can be calibrated quite easily as long as there is access to either a densitometer, an already calibrated step wedge or a pre-exposed step wedge film of known log It exposures.

With the calibrated step wedge in position and a piece of lead rubber covering an area on the film equal to the size of the uncalibrated step wedge, an exposure is made.

The uncalibrated step wedge is then placed on what was the covered area and lead rubber is used to cover all other portions of the same film. Another exposure is now made. The film is then processed.

A characteristic curve is then drawn from the results obtained from the calibrated step wedge. The density values produced by the *uncalibrated* step wedge are now measured.

Intercepts are drawn from each of these density values to the curve and then to the log It axis. These log It values represent the actual values for this step wedge at the kV selected (Fig. 8.6).

Densitometers

Densitometers read the relative density of the various steps on the film by measuring the quantity of light which passes through an area. The more light that passes through, the lower the density. This information can either be directly read off the LED display for each step and then the characteristic curve plotted by hand; or, in the more sophisticated models, the densitometer can be linked to a computer. All the steps are automatically read, and the quality control information can be automatically printed along with the characteristic curve for the film. In addition, information can be stored and weekly or monthly printouts produced if required to show the trends in processor activity and to allow comparisons between various processors that a department may have.

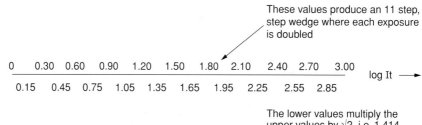

Fig. 8.5 Log It scale, calibrated for both 11 and 21 step wedge.

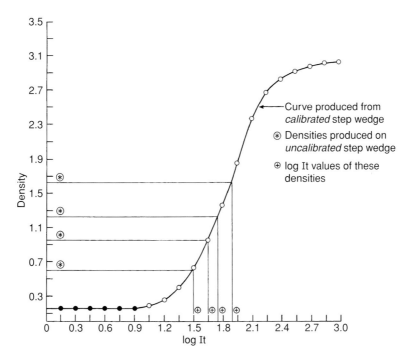

Fig. 8.6 Density values produced by uncalibrated step wedge measured against characteristic curve produced from calibrated step wedge, giving log It values of those densities.

INFORMATION FROM THE CHARACTERISTIC CURVE

A great deal of information can be gained from the characteristic curve. The main areas, illustrated in Figure 8.7, are as follows:

1. From 0 to point 1, *Basic fog*.
2. Point A, *Threshold*.
3. From A to B, the *Toe*.
4. From point B to C, the *Straight line portion*.
5. The area around D, the *Shoulder*.
6. Point E, *Maximum density*.
7. From F onwards, the *Region of solarisation*.

Basic fog (from 0 to 1)

This section of the curve is often referred to as 'base plus fog' or 'basic fog' (either version is correct).

> **The recorded density of the base, which may be tinted blue for example, plus the recorded density of the chemical fog which may have built up in the emulsion during storage, processing, etc.**

An overall increase in basic fog can affect many other measurements on the characteristic curve. There are three main categories of faults causing fog:

1. Faults that can occur in storage
2. Faults that can occur in the department or darkroom
3. Faults that occur in processing.

Storage faults

- *Too long a time in storage*
  All films have a shelf life. Increased storage time allows chemical fog to build up to sometimes unacceptable levels.

- *Temperature too high*
  About 10°C is required for prolonged storage. High temperatures accelerate the ageing process.

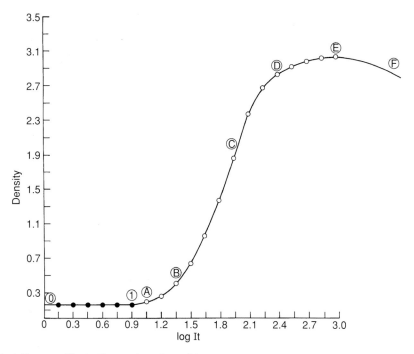

Fig. 8.7 Characteristic curve, illustrating main points of interest.

- *Humidity too high*
  The relative humidity should be 50%. High humidity, in unprotected boxes, can lead to the film continuing ripening while in storage.

- *Films stored horizontally*
  Films should be stored vertically. If they are stored horizontally then pressure marks are inevitably created on the lowest films.

- *High background radiation*
  The effect of background radiation leads to a linear increase in basic fog.

- *Fumes*
  A great many fumes can fog film. They are almost too numerous to mention, but a few examples are carbon monoxide, certain paint fumes, formalin, formaldehyde and mercury vapour.

- *Scattered radiation*
  It is wise to keep a film store well away from an X-ray room, even if the protection is considered adequate.

Darkroom faults

Many sources of fogging can be found in a darkroom, many of them connected with safelights.

- *Incorrect safelight*
  If an orange filter is used with orthochromatic film, the film will fog on exposure to the safelight. There is a simple way of remembering safelight colours (Fig. 8.8). The safest separation should always be two colours away from the maximum sensitivity of the film.

- *Too long handling time*
  See Safelight test, p. 201.

- *Too many safelights*
  No explanation is really needed. See Safelight test, p. 201.

- *Safelights too close*
  About 1 m is the closest that should be considered.

- *Too bright safelights*
  With a tungsten bulb in the safelight, the maximum wattage should be 25 W.

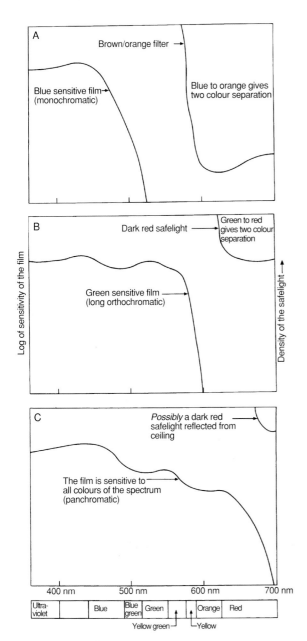

Fig. 8.8 Determining correct safelight colours.

- *Cracked safelights*
  A regular check of safelights will obviate this problem.
- *Light leakage*
  White light of low intensity striking the film in a darkroom can produce an overall fog.

Processing faults

For detailed references to these faults see Processor evaluation, pp. 193–9.

- *Over-replenishment*
  Over-replenishment causes unselectivity of the exposed and unexposed silver halide grains.

- *Too high developer temperature*
  Again, this causes unselectivity.

- *Too long a processing time*
  Again, causes unselectivity. No developer is totally selective, all developers will eventually develop every silver halide grain.

- *Contamination*
  If developer is contaminated by fixer, then basic fog will begin to rise. Eventually, an overall grey film will result, with a density around 1.0. Long before this happens there will be a smell of ammonia. This is the *only* time in the photographic process when ammonia can be smelt. The only action that can be taken is to drain the developer tank, wash it out thoroughly and start again. Note that fixer contamination of developer can be measured in parts per million.

Fixer

It is also important to remember that fixer can cause an overall increase in basic fog:

- *Temperature*
  Fixing time is directly related to the temperature of the fixer. If the fixer becomes too cold, perhaps because a heater has broken down in the processor, the film may be only partially fixed. This can result in an overall fog on the film. Of course, the film will not store for a long period and the image will deteriorate rapidly.

- *Time*
  If a film is in the fixer for too short a time, the result will be exactly as listed under fixer temperature.

- *Under-replenishment*
  This causes non-fixation of the film. The results are identical to those listed under fixer temperature.

It will be seen that increases in basic fog play a very important part in the characteristic curve, as it affects many of the measurements made.

Threshold (point A) and toe (point A to B)

A film could be exposed to an amount of radiation as measured on the log It axis and still show no response.

> **Threshold is the point at which the film first shows a reaction to exposure.**

This has a relevance in safelight testing, where the film has to receive a 'flash exposure' to take the film past threshold, before commencing the test. This explains why film is so much more sensitive to mishandling after exposure, i.e. after it has been sensitised. The toe is an area of rapidly increasing gradient.

The straight line portion (from B to C)

When looking closely at the curve (see Fig. 8.7) it can be seen that there is no 'straight line' portion. The curve on medical X-ray screen film resembles more of an elongated 'S'. However, the name remains and it is this section of the characteristic curve which carries a very large amount of information on:

- Gamma
- Contrast
- Average gradient
- Useful exposure range
- Useful density range
- Film latitude
- Speed.

Gamma and its other derivatives

Looking at Figure 8.9, consider the derivation of the tangent of angle A.

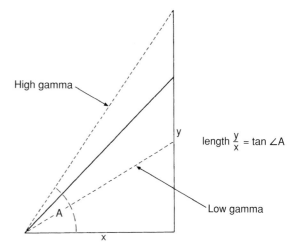

Fig. 8.9 Determining Gamma.

$$\left[\frac{\text{Opposite}}{\text{Adjacent}}\right] = \frac{\text{Side } y}{\text{Side } x} = \text{Tangent of angle A}$$

If this triangle is superimposed over the characteristic curve in the region of the straight line portion, it can be seen that a measurement of the slope of the curve can be made.

Contrast

It is important to appreciate that the angle of this slope, when expressed as a tangent, is exactly equal in numerical terms to the Gamma. It also follows that the larger the angle (i.e. the steeper the slope), the higher the Gamma. This means, in photographic terms, that the film will have a higher contrast (and so will look 'black and white'). The exact opposite is also true: the smaller the angle, the less steep the slope, the lower the overall contrast (and so will have more 'shades of grey').

If there had been a true straight line section, the triangle could have been superimposed exactly. Unfortunately, on medical X-ray screen film there is no straight line, and therefore an estimate has to be made of where the straight line portion is. This will vary from individual to individual. An estimate is clearly unsatisfactory, and so a better method has to be used.

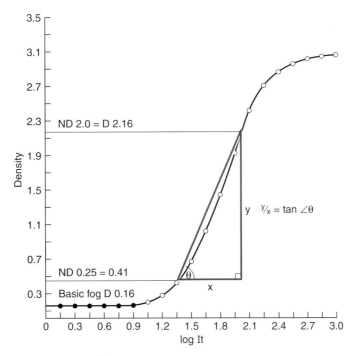

Fig. 8.10 Determining average gradient (G̅).

Average gradient (or average Gamma)

This is usually denoted by G̅.

To calculate the average gradient, a triangle is constructed using defined points, *net density* 0.25 and *net density* 2.0 (Fig. 8.10). With this measurement of the slope we gain the true value of the *average* contrast available in the straight line portion of the characteristic curve.

What is net density? Net density is the density required plus basic fog.

What amount of energy is required to raise this film to net density 1? If one film has a basic fog of 0.6 and another film has one of 0.18, unless net density was used the first film would appear to be much faster (Fig. 8.11).

Why are 0.25 and 2.0 chosen as the points on the curve to establish average gradient? Only 1.0% of the incident light reaches the viewer's eye at density 2. On the average viewing box there is not enough light emitted to penetrate through density 2. Hence the choice of density 2.

Why 0.25? The higher the slope of the curve the higher the contrast, the lower the slope the lower the contrast. If an average value is taken of the contrast available in the toe of the curve it will be extremely low indeed. As the eye can only discern differences in contrast of about 10%

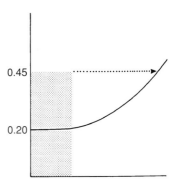

Fig. 8.11 Net density is that density which the film achieves solely by actinic radiation. Therefore, when determining a net density the amount of basic fog present on the film must be taken into account. The basic fog present is 0.20; the net density required is 0.25. The basic fog and the net density are added (0.20 + 0.25) and the measurement is made at 0.45.

it becomes obvious that there is simply insufficient contrast available much below net density 0.25. Hence the choice of 0.25. These are also the values of the maximum and minimum useful densities.

Variants

The two points used to measure average gradient mentioned will vary with the type of material used, as the curves will vary considerably according to film type. The following film types require the different values shown, to measure average gradient:

Cinefluorography	0.25 and 1.25 + basic fog
Image intensifier	0.25 and 1.75 + basic fog
Monitor photography	0.25 and 1.75 + basic fog
Photofluorography	0.25 and 2.0 + basic fog
Film/screen techniques	0.25 and 2.0 + basic fog

In summary

1. The tangent of the angle the slope makes is numerically equal to the average gradient.

2. The value of this tangent tells us the average value of contrast available within the straight line portion.

3. The steeper the slope, the higher the contrast and vice versa.

4. Two points are used to construct the triangle, net density 0.25 and net density 2.0 for screen films.

Image contrast = subject contrast × average gradient

The above formula indicates that the final contrast seen on the film is a result of the initial subject contrast multiplied by the average gradient. Consider the two films in Figure 8.12. With an average gradient of 2.5 for film A (a good average value), there is an amplification of the subject contrast by a factor of 2.5.

Subject contrast is very difficult to arrive at absolutely and some explanation may be necessary. It means that a curve has to be drawn and then the maximum and minimum values of mAs (as log It values) passing through the body areas are assessed. The intercepts are then drawn from

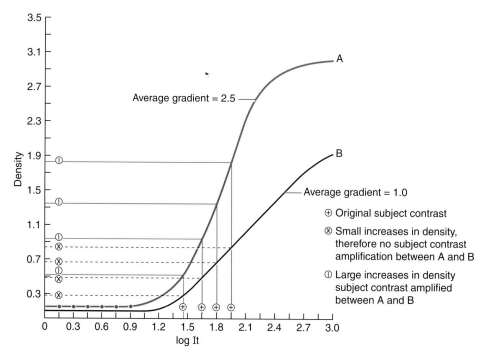

Fig. 8.12 Average gradient for two films, showing potential effect of amplification of subject contrast.

these points to the curve and then to the density axis. With an average gradient of 2.5, large increases of density are produced, *in the region of useful exposure*, for relatively low increases in exposure.

With a very low average gradient of 1.0 with film B (which incidentally is an unusable value in medical radiography), the image contrast is equal to the subject contrast, no amplification of contrast is possible. Now only small increases in density are produced for the same increases in exposure as were used with film A.

The value of the average gradient is not the only information which can be gained from this section of the curve. Information on the useful exposure range, speed and latitude is readily available.

Useful exposure and density range

If the full characteristic curve is constructed and then two vertical lines drawn from the intercepts of the two net densities, the useful exposure range for the film can then be determined.

In the case of Figure 8.13, the log It axis of the curve is intercepted at 1.36 and 2.05. If this axis is considered as a log relative exposure axis, the figures will seem to be fairly arbitrary. It becomes clearer if the log It axis is considered to be the *absolute* value of mAs at a certain kV and that these values have been used to plot the curve. Incidentally, the mAs values were obtained by taking antilogs of each log It value on the scale.

Absolute values as an example

log It 0	=	1 mAs
log It 0.30	=	2 mAs
log It 0.60	=	4 mAs
log It 0.90	=	8 mAs
log It 1.20	=	16 mAs
log It 1.50	=	32 mAs
log It 1.80	=	64 mAs
log It 2.10	=	128 mAs
log It 2.40	=	256 mAs
log It 2.70	=	512 mAs
log It 3.00	=	1024 mAs

Note that these values have been taken as actual mAs values of log It. However, the

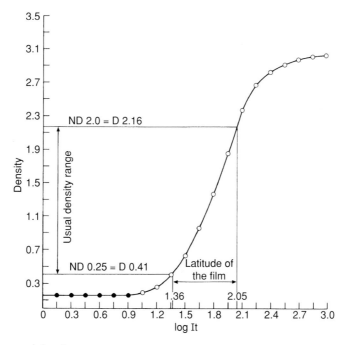

Fig. 8.13 Usual exposure and density range.

relationship between exposures for these log It values always remain the same.

As these values are now assumed to be the *actual* mAs values at a certain kV, the useful range of exposures would be between 23 and 112 mAs at that particular kV.

These figures were obtained by finding the antilog of 1.36 and 2.05 respectively. On the scale showing actual mAs values as an example, 1.36 will equal 23 mAs and 2.05 will equal 112 mAs.

Below an exposure of 23 mAs actually reaching the film, a very low density film would be obtained. Above 112 mAs reaching the film, a very black film would be obtained. Both of these exposures would not utilise the film correctly. In the first example, exposures will have been made in the toe area of the curve, whereas in the second example, exposures were made in the shoulder. In both cases, the exposures would have been made outside the straight line portion of the curve. It might therefore be better to consider that the straight line portion is more correctly named 'the region of useful exposure'. This exposure latitude is irrevocably linked to the average gradient of the film. The higher the average gradient, the lower the latitude of the film. The lower the average gradient, the higher the latitude.

This knowledge is particularly useful when setting up automatic exposure devices so that they can be triggered to stop when the exposure has reached the mid-point of the curve. Usually, however, the log It axis is used merely to refer to the relationship between the exposures. For example, starting with 6 mAs as log It 0, then log It 1.20 will be 96 mAs, etc.

This figure is obtained as follows:

log It 0   = 6 mAs
log It 0.3 = 12 mAs
log It 0.6 = 24 mAs
log It 0.9 = 48 mAs
log It 1.2 = 96 mAs

Similar relationships exist across the log It scale. It only means remembering that log It 0.3 is equal to doubling (or halving) the exposure.

It can be seen from the above explanations that only in the region of useful exposure are almost linear gains made in density increase. Below the

intercept from net density 0.25, there are small or non-existent gains in density. Above the intercept of net density 2.0, similar small gains are made for the same increase in exposure. It is only in the useful range of exposures that large density gains are made *for the same increases in exposure* (Fig. 8.14).

Latitude of the film

The region of useful exposure can be used to define the latitude of the film. Looking at Figure 8.13 we can see the useful exposure range which will also tell us the amount of under- or over-exposure the film will tolerate.

Speed

If a 35 mm film is purchased for a camera, it is easy to determine the speed of the film by the ISO number: the higher the number, the faster the film. This is not so easy with X-ray film.

To define the speed of an X-ray film can sometimes be difficult. Consider the curves illustrated in Figure 8.15. Note that two of these films (C and A) are unusable in an X-ray department as screen films. Film C has an unusable latitude, and film A has an average gradient of 1.0 (see under Variants, p. 160). Films B and D are almost identical, apart from speed differences.

One film must be faster than another, if it reaches a certain density with a lower exposure than the other film. Considering films B and C, film C is the fastest film because it reached density 1 well before film B. However, films A and D create a different problem. A is faster than D below density 1.35, and slower than D above density 1.35.

It is usual to say that the further over to the left the curve lies, the faster the film. In the case of films A and D it has to be qualified, by adding 'above or below a certain density'.

In the ANSI (American National Standards Institute) specifications, X-ray film speed is defined as the exposure required for the film to reach net density 1 (Fig. 8.16).

If this fact is now transferred to Figure 8.15, it can be seen that:

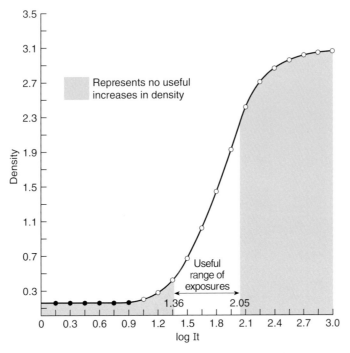

Fig. 8.14 Small increases in exposure in the useful exposure range will increase density appreciably; above net density 2.0 and below net density 0.25, only small or non-existent gains in density are made for the same increases.

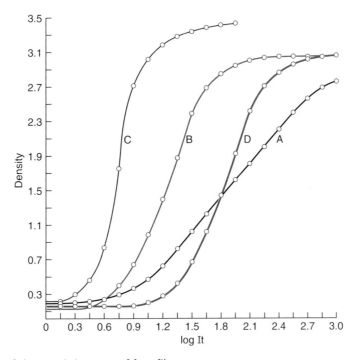

Fig. 8.15 Comparison of characteristic curves of four films.

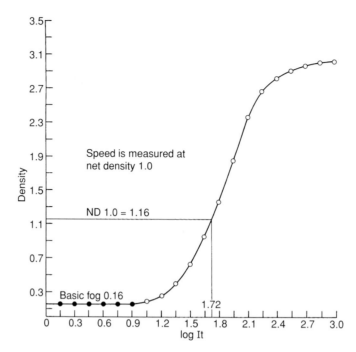

Fig. 8.16 Film speed is measured at net density 1.0.

Film A has a speed of log It 1.67
Film B has a speed of log It 1.14
Film C has a speed of log It 0.68
Film D has a speed of log It 1.73.

This fact can be extremely useful when films are being compared using an accurate exposure device. It provides a very accurate figure which can be expressed in percentage terms (e.g. 25% faster) or in log It exposure differences. For example, if full sensitometric curves are produced, the speed of both films may be measured and compared, as shown in Figure 8.17.

In this case the films are separated by a log It difference of log It 0.3. This means that film X is 100% faster than film Y (i.e. film Y requires twice the exposure of film X) or, within the range 50–80 kV, there is a 10 kV difference in speed. Thus, absolute values can be found for differences in film speed.

When speed comparisons are made in the imaging department, the measurements are usually comparative. In this case the two films to be tested are placed in the same cassette and an exposure is made through a step wedge. (It is not necessary for this wedge to be calibrated.) The film producing the highest density at the same step is the fastest.

A similar type of test can also be used to compare screens. In this case the step wedge exposure would be made on the two cassettes to be tested, ideally with the wedge covering the two cassettes so that only the one exposure is required. The films may then be compared in the way described above for density differences. Complete sensitometry can be undertaken and very accurate figures obtained by measuring the actual log It differences.

Shoulder (area around point D)

The point at which the film's reaction to exposure begins to fall off.

In the straight line portion of the curve, large increases in density were achieved by relatively small increases in exposure.

In the shoulder of the curve, the density increases are very small indeed for the same increases in exposure. Eventually, the curve begins to flatten completely and it is at this point that D max, or maximum density, is reached.

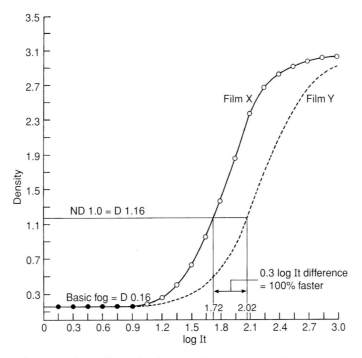

Fig. 8.17   Full sensitometric curves of two films, allowing speed to be compared.

Maximum density (point E)

The maximum density which can be reached on the film, under this set of exposure and processing conditions.

This is often referred to as Max D, or D max.

Region of solarisation (point F onwards)

The point at which the density on the film begins to decrease for increases in exposure, i.e. a reversal image can be obtained.

To reach this area on the film a large amount of overexposure is required, usually of the order of several thousands of times.

It is caused by the silver halide grain not being able to absorb any more energy and the grain beginning to re-associate into the silver bromide, instead of breaking down into silver and bromine ions.

Solarisation is sometimes observed on X-ray films in the department. It is safe to say it is never caused by direct overexposure, but may be the result of prolonged exposure to safelight after exposure in the X-ray room.

The phenomenon of solarisation is used in the manufacture of copying films. In this case the desired effect is that the film should react so that any light areas are produced as light areas and dark areas as dark. If ordinary X-ray film was used to make a copy, the light areas would be reproduced as dark areas. When the film is manufactured as a solarised film, presolarisation is usually produced by chemical means.

SPEED VERSUS DEFINITION

This section of the text should be read in conjunction with Chapter 9, Image quality, as the information in that chapter is apposite to the area under discussion. In Chapter 9, reference is made to the way in which the image quality can be affected by a change in the speed of the film. The illustrations of the arrowhead (Fig. 9.11) explain in detail how the resolution, and hence the image quality, can be altered. The essential conclusion arrived at is that the faster the film, the worse the definition (this, of course, implies the use of similar emulsions).

Quantum mottle

Much has been written about quantum mottle, which is really a phenomenon which interferes with diagnosis and appears as marked 'graininess' on the film. It is directly related to the dose (mAs) reaching the film (i.e. the lower the dose, the higher the quantum mottle, and vice versa).

It should be said that the illustrations for quantum mottle were produced using a random number generator to position the 'quanta'. On a macroscopic scale it could be said that they fairly represent actuality.

In Figure 8.18 the dots represent X-ray quanta arriving at the film. The figure also illustrates the perfect world, which of course does not exist. X-ray quanta do not arrive evenly at the film, but vary randomly over the film surface. Nevertheless, the shape of an 'X' can be clearly seen.

Figure 8.19 represents reality. Exactly the same number of quanta are present, but they are now striking the film randomly. Statistically, with high levels of irradiation the quanta are scattered fairly evenly over the film surface. Because of this high level of irradiation, the image can still be clearly seen.

With half the exposure, only half the quanta are available (Fig. 8.20). Now the image is not clearly rendered, as the randomness of the quanta landing produces marked variations of density over the film. The dose is now so low that the film begins to record individual quanta and the apparent 'grain' (the record of the single quantum) begins to appear.

Exposures can be so low that only individual quanta will be recorded, insufficient even to record an image. It has been suggested by many sources that quantum mottle is the factor which limits the ultimate speed of any film/screen system.

Quantum mottle, therefore, has an effect similar to an increase of film speed, in that it reduces the ultimate definition of the system by increased graininess. The effects of both the speed of the film and quantum mottle are similar, but the causes are very different.

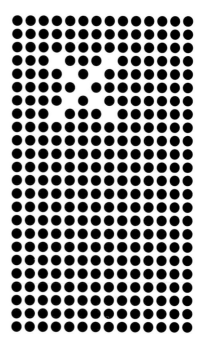

Fig. 8.18 X-ray quanta striking film (theoretical representation).

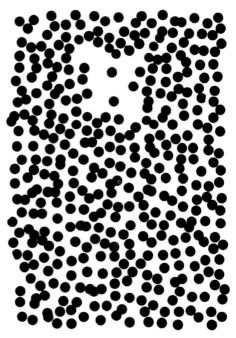

Fig. 8.19 X-ray quanta striking film (representation of reality, with quanta striking film randomly).

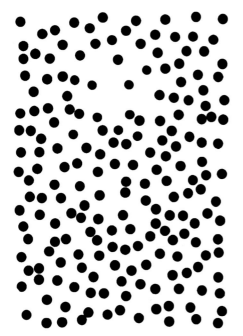

Fig. 8.20 X-ray quanta striking film, half exposure of Fig. 8.19.

CONCLUSIONS

Sensitometry is a part of photography which, if well understood, can give the user a great deal of information about the behaviour of film, screens and the automatic processor within the department. It also plays a major part in a quality assurance programme (see Ch. 10).

The principal uses of sensitometry are:

1. To compare different *types of film*.
2. To compare different *types of screens*.
3. As a useful tool for setting up *exposure devices*.
4. To determine *average gradient*, and therefore subject contrast amplification.
5. To find *film and exposure latitude*.
6. To find the absolute value of the *speed of films*.
7. To *monitor* the performance of an *automatic processor*.

Note:

The characteristic curve is only valid under a certain set of processing conditions.

Any alteration of processing conditions in terms of speed of throughput, changes in temperature, changes in chemistry, etc., can drastically alter any results.

Chapter 9
Image quality

CHAPTER CONTENTS

INTRODUCTION

The radiologist or clinician requires the highest quality images available to enable the most accurate diagnosis and treatment. It is the radiographer's job to produce those images.

To identify a high quality image is not easy. In the following pages an attempt has been made to lead the reader through the subject of assessing image quality. Frequent reference will be made to other topics more fully covered by other chapters.

SIGNAL TO NOISE RATIO

Image quality may be defined as the signal to noise ratio:

$$\text{Image quality} = \frac{\text{signal}}{\text{noise}}$$

- The signal is the information required from the imaging system, e.g. the radiograph
- The signal can be defined as the minimum size of the object that must be visible
- The noise is anything that may detract from that signal
- The noise, in the conventional film/screen system, could be defined as the graininess of the image.

The formula may be used to assess image quality in any system, providing the signal and noise can be measured.

If the signal level is very high the object will be clearly seen, but if the signal level is similar to the noise level, the object will be very difficult to see, as it will be partially obliterated by the noise. A simple analogy is the television system. With the old 405 line transmitters, scattered over quite wide distances, there was very often 'snow' visible on the TV picture (i.e. a low signal : noise ratio). With the improved 625 line transmitters, usually covering a small area, the picture is considerably improved. In other words, the signal : noise ratio has been increased. The remainder of this chapter is concerned with assessing the photographic quality of a conventional film/screen image.

Looking at Figure 9.1, if the sharpness of the system is increased the visually disturbing noise will also increase, as now the system is resolving the noise better as well as giving a sharper signal. If the contrast is increased the signal will appear to be clearer, but so will the noise. It is impossible to compensate for all the factors, and therefore the final result has to be a compromise.

RESOLUTION AND MODULATION TRANSFER FUNCTION

Sharpness, or resolution, is measured using a line pair (lp) phantom. The line pair phantom is made up of strips of lead separated by an air gap equal to the width of the preceding lead strip. Starting at low frequencies (perhaps 1 line pair per millimetre, or lp mm^{-1}), the phantom then progressively decreases the width of the lead strip and the following air gap until high frequencies, perhaps as high as 10 or 14 lp mm^{-1}, are reached (Fig. 9.2).

Resolution

Resolution can be defined as:

The size of the smallest object or distance between two objects that must exist before the imaging system will record that object or objects as separate entities.

It gives no indication of how the system will record objects of larger dimensions or whether they will be visible to an observer. Usually measured in line pairs per millimetre (lp mm^{-1}), resolution has a limited value in assessing system

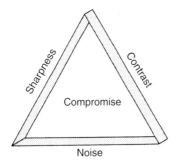

Fig. 9.1 Image quality is a compromise between sharpness, contrast and noise.

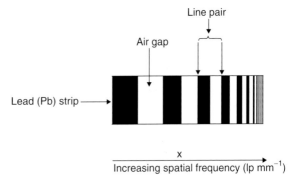

Fig. 9.2 Example of one type of line pair phantom.

performance. Definition is a subjective impression of the details that can be seen in the radiograph and is difficult to quantify and should not be confused with resolution.

Modulation transfer function (MTF)

This allows assessment of system performance at different spatial frequencies (i.e. 'object sizes'). It would be expected that the differences in density of the line pair phantom would be recorded in exactly the same way as the original phantom with the sharp edges clearly delineated, as illustrated in Figure 9.3.

Because of transition density within the film, distinct transition edges are formed which produce a density reading similar to the one in Figure 9.4 when scanned with a microdensitometer.

It can be seen that at low frequencies the transfer of the signal through the system is quite good. As the frequencies get higher the contrast begins to drop rapidly and the pairs of lines become impossible to see.

If a number of calculations are done, figures can be obtained for the percentage of accuracy of the transfer of the signal through the system. In this way the modulation, or altering, of the signal through the system is measured and the modulation transfer function (MTF) for the system has been obtained (Fig. 9.5).

The *degree* of sharpness required, however, raises many questions.

Illustrated in Figure 9.6 are four different films, each with markedly different MTF characteristics. It would appear at first glance that film A is the one that should be chosen for work in a general radiographic department, as this transfers most information at low and high frequencies.

EFFECT OF SCREENS

Now consider Figure 9.7. It is generally accepted that in a general radiographic department, the maximum resolution required is about

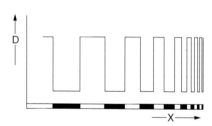

Fig. 9.3 Reading from an image of a perfectly transferred line pair phantom (100% transfer at all frequencies).

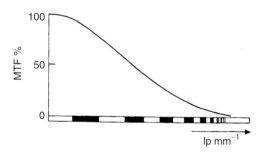

Fig. 9.5 Example of MTF curve, showing loss of information transfer at high spatial frequencies, e.g. at high lp mm^{-1}.

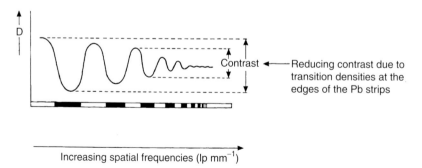

Fig. 9.4 Example of an actual density profile obtained from a line pair phantom showing decreasing information transfer at higher lp mm^{-1}, owing to transition densities.

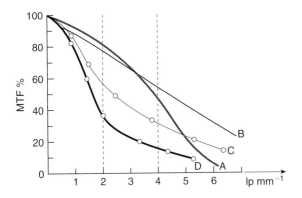

Fig. 9.6 Example of four different MTF curves.

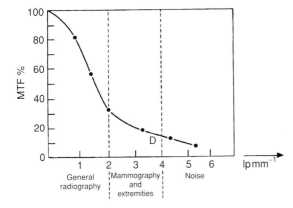

Fig. 9.7 Suggested limiting resolutions shown on an MTF curve (curve D from Fig. 9.6).

2 lp mm^{-1}. For *mammography*, for example, the demands are greater, and perhaps 4 lp mm^{-1} are required. The minimum size of object it is required to see has now been defined (i.e. the signal). Therefore, everything smaller than this size is information that is not required and is considered noise (Fig. 9.7).

Now consider how an intensifying screen achieves its efficiency.

$$\text{Total \% efficiency} = \text{absorption \%} \times \text{conversion \%}$$

In every case it is better to go for a high absorption of the *image forming quanta* than to rely on conversion to gain speed, as this reduces the noise.

Consider Figure 9.8. All of the screens in Figure 9.8 are class 200 and yet they achieve their total efficiency in many different ways. The best choice for image quality would be screen 6. This would be the sharpest, as it has the lowest quantum mottle (because of its high absorption) and the lowest lateral light scatter, because of the dye tint.

Having now established the construction of the screen and its ultimate sharpness, more questions can be raised:

- Should the phosphors be conventional calcium tungstate?
- Should the phosphors be rare earth?
- Should the phosphors emit green, blue or UV light?

The question of which phosphors to use is complex and requires a fairly detailed explanation.

Calcium tungstate is an established phosphor and with modern coating techniques can be a very useful phosphor in a range of intensifying screens.

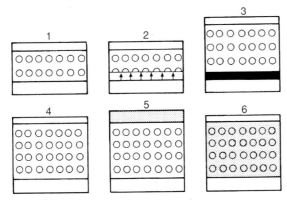

	Absorption	Conversion
1	Reference	Reference
2	Low	High
3	High	Low
4	High	Low
5	High	Low
6	High	Low

Fig. 9.8 Six different screen constructions, all with the same speed class. Which produces the best image quality?

The absorption efficiency of the rare earth phosphors is at least 50% better than calcium tungstate. Conversion efficiency is at least four times better than calcium tungstate. Thus, the total efficiency of a rare earth system is many times better than calcium tungstate. The *advantages of rare earth phosphors are:*

1. They offer decreased radiation exposure to both staff and patients

2. There is reduced movement unsharpness, as shorter exposure times are usually available

3. There can be reduced geometric unsharpness as longer focus film distances can be used without an increase in exposure

4. There will be lower tube loadings

5. There is the availability to use fine focus more often, again decreasing geometric unsharpness

6. There is the ability to use grids with a higher grid ratio, thereby producing better quality images

7. It is possible to produce increased contrast, by reducing the kV instead of the mAs.

When film/screen combinations are first designed there are a number of image quality parameters to take into account. They are, *contrast, sharpness* and *noise*: the compromise needed between them was mentioned at the beginning of this chapter.

Statements are made about the benefits or otherwise of green or blue/UV-emitting systems, many without scientific foundation.

- Films can be made to virtually any reasonable sensitometric profile: therefore, in terms of contrast, orthochromatic and monochromatic films can be identical.

- When sharpness is considered, two factors, crossover and phosphor, need to be mentioned.

Crossover

Film acts as a natural absorber for UV and blue light. Therefore, crossover in both of these systems is low, for blue less than 50%. In the UV systems it can be as low as 20%, which is negligible.

In orthochromatic systems, crossover is much higher unless the film is specially treated. Crossover can be measured as high as 70%, which leads to a less sharp image.

It can be said that, in terms of sharpness caused by crossover, the UV/blue-emitting systems are better.

Phosphor

Table 9.1 lists the varying characteristics of three rare earth screen systems. The UV-emitting barium fluorochloride screen (BaFCl) reaches its efficiency by having absorption and conversion in the correct ratios. Because of the very low crossover associated with UV, this screen is eminently suitable for very fast systems.

Gadolinium oxysulphide ($Gd_2O_2S_2$) gains its efficiency by its higher conversion, relative to lanthanum oxybromide (LaOBr). This would lead to greater unsharpness, as it is higher absorption that always leads to better sharpness and image quality. However, as the specific weight of gadolinium is greater than lanthanum, the coating weight can be less. The gadolinium screen can be made thinner, thus leading to better sharpness. Therefore, overall, the systems are virtually equal in performance, although there

Table 9.1 Characteristics of different phosphors			
Characteristics	Ortho ($Gd_2O_2S_2$)	Blue (LaOBr)	UV (BaFCl)
% Absorption 80 kV	40.5	43.5	39.0
% Conversion	18.0	17.0	16.0
Specific weight	7.4	6.2	4.6
Phosphor thickness (μ)	207	228	347
Efficiency	7.3	7.4	6.2

might be a preference for the monochromatic system, as silver halide is naturally sensitive to UV and blue light and therefore does not have to be sensitised. Also, no special darkroom lighting is required.

EFFECT OF FILM

Most manufacturers produce both full and half speed film.

Half speed film really came into being with the emergence of rare earth phosphors. The film was necessary, particularly with the very fast systems, as it markedly reduced quantum mottle. There was also another reason: the image quality improved when this film was used.

The following example explains why the combination of a slow film and a fast screen helps to produce high quality images (Table 9.2). Note, the numbers of quanta are examples only and realistically they should be raised by many powers.

System A is a monochromatic film and blue-emitting screens. If 100 X-ray quanta are required to produce a density of 1 on the film. In Table 9.2 column one, 20 original information-carrying X-ray quanta have been absorbed, producing 1000 light photons to give the film to density 1.0.

System B (Table 9.2 column two) would require exactly half the exposure of system A. Special screens require only half the exposure of the universal screens, hence only 50 X-ray quanta are needed. However, because special screens have an absorption of 40%, 20 quanta are absorbed, exactly the same number as universal screens.

System C (Table 9.2 column three) reverts to a class 100 system, using special screens and a

half speed film. The system becomes half speed, and requires 100 X-ray quanta again. Because a special screen is used, 40 information-carrying quanta are absorbed. These absorbed quanta produce 2000 light photons and, because it is a half speed film, raise it to density 1.

Therefore, in system A only 20 of the information-carrying quanta are absorbed (in other words, over 80 of these quanta are not used).

The easiest way to increase the absorption of the screens would be to substitute a faster screen, which must be able to absorb more quanta, as the usual way to increase screen speed is to increase the coating thickness of the phosphor.

In system B exactly the same number of quanta are absorbed because, although the number of X-ray quanta is halved, the absorption is doubled.

In system C, 40 of the information-carrying quanta are absorbed and only 60 are lost. Therefore high quality/low noise images can be produced using half speed film.

The above arguments would also hold true for orthochromatic systems.

CONTRAST

A radiograph is the product of a transfer of information. During this transfer it is exposed to a number of different influences. Contrast goes a long way to determining the quality of the radiograph. There are four principal types of contrast:

- Subject contrast
- Film contrast
- Radiographic contrast
- Subjective contrast.

Table 9.2 Comparison of three film/screen systems

	System A	System B	System C
Number of X-ray quanta	100	50	100
Type of screen	Universal	Special	Universal
Percentage absorption	20%	40%	40%
Photons emitted	1000	1000	2000
Film type	Normal	Normal	Half speed
Net density	1.0	1.0	1.0

Subject contrast

This is caused by differential attenuation and absorption of the X-ray beam as it passes through the patient (i.e. the subject). It is responsible for the differing intensities of the emergent X-ray beam, and therefore the exposures that eventually reach the film. Figure 9.9 represents the same thickness of bone and fatty tissue. The bone attenuates more of the beam than the fatty tissue and therefore the emergent intensity in the area below the bone is less than the surrounding fatty tissue. The film receives less exposure and produces a lower photographic density when compared to the fatty tissue areas. In this case the subject contrast can be defined as the ratio of the emergent intensities, i.e.:

$$\text{Subject contrast} = \frac{1_F}{1_B}$$

The factors affecting subject contrast are:

- Different thicknesses of the same tissue
- Different densities of the same tissue
- Different atomic numbers of the tissues
- Radiation quality (kVp, anode material, etc.)
- Use of contrast agents.

Different thicknesses

Consider two different thicknesses of the same tissue type. The thicker of the two will attenuate more of the beam and allow less exposure to reach

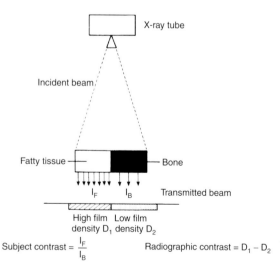

Fig. 9.9 Diagrammatic illustration of subject contrast.

the film. Subject contrast is the ratio of the intensity that has passed through the thin part, compared to the thicker part.

Different densities

Consider the same tissue with the same volume but at a higher density (i.e. higher mass per unit volume). The higher density will attenuate more of the beam. This will reduce the intensity of the emergent beam and thus affect the subject contrast.

Different atomic numbers

The higher the atomic number of a substance, the higher the attenuation of the incident X-ray beam. At the energies used in diagnostic radiography, photoelectric absorption predominates and is the largest contributing factor to subject contrast.

Radiation quality

In this case, radiation quality means the kilovoltage (kV) set for the exposure. For the same subject, increasing the kV decreases the difference in intensities of the emergent beam and therefore decreases the subject contrast. Low kV will produce high subject contrast, but the kV must be high enough to adequately penetrate the area being examined.

Also:

- Changing kV gives a high contrast variation in bone work
- The influence of kV is smaller on soft tissue rendition
- In the low kV range, 10 kV has more effect on contrast than in the higher kV range
- In the middle kV range, 20 kV is needed to give an appreciable change in contrast.

Other factors also determine the radiation quality and therefore the final subject contrast. There are:

- The anode material, e.g. mammography
- Varying voltage ripple components
- Tube filters and supplementary filters
- Scattered radiation.

The anode material, voltage components and tube filtration are determined by the X-ray equipment in use.

The influence of scatter is mainly felt in two ways:

- Radiation fog, which increases the overall photographic density of the film
- Reduction in the image latitude.

Limiting these effects is of prime importance if high quality images are to be obtained. In general the higher the selected kV, the higher the amount of scatter and the higher the radiation fog and reduction in image latitude. However, as previously stated, the kV must be high enough to penetrate the area being examined. Therefore the use of grids, collimators, compression bands and other methods of reducing the production of scatter should always be considered.

Use of contrast agents

These may be positive agents (e.g. non-ionic iodine compounds or barium) or negative agents (e.g. carbon dioxide or air). In either case, they are normally used to fill a cavity or space in the body that usually has a low subject contrast when compared to surrounding structures. The agent alters the subject contrast by either increasing the X-ray absorption properties of the structure concerned, or decreasing the absorption

properties, with an effect on the intensity of the emergent beam. They can also be used in combination, for example double contrast barium meals and enemas.

Film and radiographic contrast

Film contrast

This is defined by the average gradient of the film (see Ch. 8, Sensitometry). It is a measure of the film's ability to amplify the subject contrast (Fig. 9.10).

Radiographic contrast

This is the photographic density difference between two adjacent areas on the film. These differences in density may or may not be observable to the naked eye.

Subjective contrast

This is the last link in the chain of contrast factors; it is the observer's opinion of the contrast that he or she sees on the film. It is a combination of all the other factors listed, plus viewing conditions, the performance of the eye, the observer's ability and, perhaps, his/her personal opinion (see Perceptibility, p. 183, and ROC, p. 184).

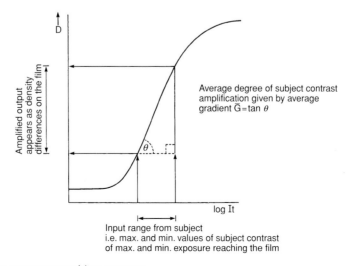

Fig. 9.10 Effect of film contrast on subject contrast.

The eye analyses the structures in the radiograph and will select details. The success rate depends on the different degrees of brightness. This ratio of difference is expressed as:

D detail – D surroundings

This variable indicates the difference in logarithmic form which suits the physiology of the eye. This measurement is also the measurement of subjective contrast, i.e.:

Contrast = D detail – D surroundings

There are other influences on contrast which must be considered:

• Viewing box and viewing conditions
• Processing conditions
• Darkroom lighting.

The importance of masking the film should be stressed. Masking improves the range in the higher densities, while reflected light and glare can seriously decrease contrast and thereby decrease the speed of perception (further details in Perceptibility, p. 183).

SUMMARY

All the contrast factors exhibited on a radiograph can dictate two important variables:

• Perceptibility
• Speed of perception.

In addition, subject contrast is initially determined by:

• kV selected
• Voltage ripple components
• Anode material
• Filtration
• Scatter
• Contrast agents.

Scatter will be reduced and contrast will be increased by:

• Collimation
• Use of grids
• Air gap technique
• Compression.

Film contrast is influenced externally by:

• Viewing box and viewing conditions
• Processing conditions
• Darkroom lighting.

Subjective contrast can be influenced by the viewing conditions themselves (see Ambient light, p. 182).

GRAININESS

Graininess is the perception of the apparent granular structure of the image (see Ch. 5, Intensifying screens). Three factors could be responsible for the apparent mottled appearance on a radiograph. These are:

1. The relatively coarse structure of the silver halide grains
2. Structure mottle
3. Quantum mottle.

Film grain

Silver halide grains in the emulsion are of microscopic size and, typically, a silver bromide crystal will be of the order of microns in size.

When the latent image is formed, the alteration to the crystal is not visible, even under an electron microscope. It is only developer that can amplify this effect.

Developer + silver bromide = an amplification factor of 10^9

After development, the exposed silver bromide crystal splits and threads of metallic silver merge with the threads of neighbouring crystals, in turn causing visible graininess. The graininess is increased as a result of the superimposition of the two emulsions. It can also be exacerbated by short development times, requiring high temperatures. In general it can be said that:

The higher the speed of the film, the greater the inherent film grain.

Consider Figure 9.11. Here an arrowhead is illustrated as the object, and represents a macroscopic view of density 1.0. A slow film (a) achieves this density by using 20 image-forming

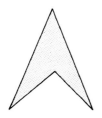 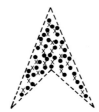

The perfect system images the 'arrowhead' perfectly with no grain. D = 1.0

(a) A 'slow' system absorbs 20 quanta → 40 developed grains → D = 1.0
Note: Some definition of arrowhead is lost

(b) A fast system. Film is now 2x the speed ∴ only 10 quanta must produce 4 developed grains per collision to reach D = 1.0. Even more definition is lost. The image is 'grainy'

x = Quanta collision
• = Developed grain

Fig. 9.11   Diagrammatic illustration of film grain in relation to film speed.

quanta and interacts with the silver halide to produce two developable grains per collision.

A film which is twice as fast (b) must necessarily use only half the number of quanta, by definition (i.e. 10 quanta). The only way that density 1.0 can be reached is by doubling the number of developable grains. Now there are four per quanta collision. Comparing the two arrowheads it is clear that (a) shows the object clearly, whereas in (b) the object is not outlined as well.

This diagram shows the effect of film grain. It should be appreciated that this effect would only be visible with significant magnification.

However, if a high speed radiographic film is exposed to *light*, grain is barely visible. It can therefore be assumed that the *largest significant factor* in the production of graininess is quantum mottle or screen mottle.

Structure mottle

This subject is fully discussed in Chapter 5, Intensifying screens, but structure mottle, particularly with modern screens, is insignificant.

Quantum mottle

When films are exposed to two different sources of energy, light only and X-radiation, the following effects occur:

Light

The energy of light is relatively low, therefore several light photons are needed to render silver bromide developable. The grain size of the film is therefore the cause of the graininess of the image.

X-radiation

The high energy of X-ray photons enables them to render a complete silver bromide crystal developable. This may require only one collision. Additionally, the production of secondary electrons by the photoelectric effect may expose neighbouring crystals, in turn rendering them developable.

The higher the energy of the radiation, the fewer photons are needed to produce a given density. Decreasing the number of quanta gives a more irregular statistical variation of the location of the quanta. This random distribution of the X-ray flux density gives the image a granular appearance which is known as quantum mottle.

Sensitivity also plays a part, as a low speed film/screen system needs a higher dose (i.e. the statistical distribution of the X-ray quanta is more even).

A formula to express this can be given as:

Quantum mottle = 1/square root of exposure

In other words, if the exposure is quadrupled the quantum mottle will be reduced by one-half.

Measurement of graininess

Graininess can be measured as density fluctuations in an area that should appear homogeneous. The measurement is made using a scanning microdensitometer.

Figure 9.12 shows the variations in readings which can be obtained with a small or large aperture. There seems to be no standard for the dimensions of the reading aperture, therefore only comparative values are possible.

$$\text{Graininess} = \theta \times \sqrt{F}$$

where

θ = variable field compensation factor
F = field size.

Graininess represents the variable noise in the system and thus is a factor affecting signal to noise ratio.

SUMMARY

- Graininess in a radiograph is chiefly a product of *exposure*.
- Graininess impairs *perception of small details* far more than large details.
- The *contrast of details* must be higher on the film if significant graininess is present.
- The largest constituent of graininess on screen film is *quantum mottle*.

- Graininess reduces *image quality* and perceptibility.

UNSHARPNESS

Unsharpness on a radiograph, photographic unsharpness (Up), is caused by the following three factors:

1. Movement of the object (Um)
2. The intensifying screens (Us)
3. The radiation geometry (Ug).

This relationship is traditionally summarised in the following formula:

$$Up = \sqrt{Um^2 + Us^2 + Ug^2}$$

although some sources suggest that the cube root of the sum of the cube of each factor should be used.

It is best if, when examining a radiograph, the major cause or causes of unsharpness are identified and reduced if possible.

Photographic unsharpness (Up)

In theory, it is quite possible to predict the expected unsharpness, but in order to do so several values must be known. For example, with a very small focal spot, large focus-film distance (ffd), no screens, an immobile object and direct exposure film the predicted result would be a

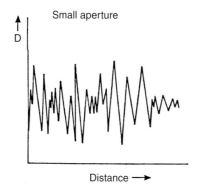

Small aperture

D

Distance →

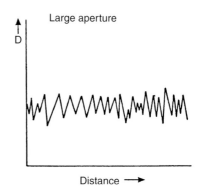

Large aperture

D

Distance →

The larger aperture evens out the density variations giving an apparently lower 'graininess'

Fig. 9.12 Density profile for the same area on a film but using a different size aperture in the microdensitometer.

sharp image. However, due to electrons released in the film and the effects of processing there will be a transition density at any edge: in other words, unsharpness.

Movement of the object (Um)

Movement unsharpness can be either voluntary or involuntary. Voluntary movement can be controlled by asking patients to hold their breath or by the use of immobilisation devices. Involuntary movement is the movement of organs or the fluid in vessels, which cannot be controlled by the patient.

Movement unsharpness (Um) is the result of the object speed (v) in any direction other than perpendicular to the film plane, in mm, multiplied by the exposure time (t) in seconds.

$$Um = v \times t$$

Strictly speaking, this value should be multiplied by the enlargement ratio, i.e. the *focus film distance* (ffd) divided by the *focus object distance* (fod). The geometric factor involved (i.e. ffd/fod) can be assumed to be about 10–20%, providing macro techniques are not used.

$$Um = v \times t \times ffd/fod$$

For example: if organ movement is about 5 mm and an exposure time of 0.2 s is used, predict the unsharpness:

$$Um = v \times t$$
$$Um = 5 \times 0.2$$
$$Um = 1 \text{ mm}$$

Therefore unsharpness = 1 mm.

If the exposure time was reduced to 0.02 s:

$$Um = v \times t$$
$$Um = 5 \times 0.02$$
$$Um = 0.1 \text{ mm}$$

Therefore unsharpness would be improved by a factor of 10.

Screen unsharpness (Us)

Screen unsharpness is influenced by the phosphor type, thickness and grain size along with the presence of an absorption/reflective layer and dye in the phosphor binder or supercoat. Full details of these are covered in Chapter 5, Intensifying screens. In addition, poor screen film contact will cause the scattering of light and therefore unsharpness; a test for screen film contact is given in Chapter 10, Quality assurance.

Quoting absolute values for screen unsharpness is difficult because so many factors are involved. Screens must reduce the sharpness of the image by the fact that light is scattered throughout the phosphor coating.

If a fast film/screen system is used to try and reduce movement unsharpness (Um), then the risk is that the inherent screen unsharpness may be greater than the reduction in Um and thus no advantage is gained. In addition, if longer exposure times are used, because of the use of lower speed screens, this could cause an increase in movement unsharpness. Therefore a compromise must always be made.

Geometric unsharpness (Ug)

This is caused by the fact that the focal spot in the tube is not a point source. Figure 9.13 shows that for a point source, the edges of an object will be recorded as sharp edges on the film. However, for an extended source, each edge of the object receives a ray as if it were two separate points, causing the penumbra effect shown, which produces unsharpness. Likewise, if the focus object distance is reduced, then the unsharpness is increased. To counter this the focus object distance needs to be increased, to reduce Ug, but this will mean increasing the mAs and perhaps the exposure time. This in turn increases Um. If the *object film distance* (ofd) is increased, Ug is increased, and an increase in exposure will be required which may increase Um. Alternatively a faster screen may be used, thus increasing Us.

For example, to calculate Ug, the ratio of the object film distance to the distance between the focal spot and the object is used. The larger the focal spot, the greater the distance between the object and the film, and the closer the focal spot is to the object, the more Ug will increase:

For example, the focus film distance (ffd) = 100 cm and the focus object distance (fod) = 80 cm.

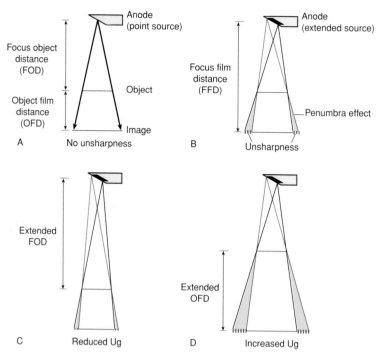

Fig. 9.13 Effect of (A) point source, (B) extended source, (C) focus object distance and (D) object film distance on geometric unsharpness (Ug).

Calculate the geometric unsharpness if a 1.2 mm focal spot was used.

$$ofd = 100 - 80 = 20 \text{ cm}$$

then

$$Ug : \text{focal spot size} = 20 : 80$$

therefore

$$Ug = 1/4 \text{ of the focal spot size.}$$

Focal spot = 1.2 mm, then

$$Ug = \frac{1.2}{4} = 0.3 \text{ mm}$$

Finally, ideally, the shortest possible exposure time, a well collimated beam, a compression band and a grid with no intensifying screens (or fine grain screens), the smallest possible focal spot, a large focus film distance, a small object film distance and, last but not least, a cooperative thin patient should produce a relatively sharp image! In reality, however, as has been illustrated, in order to achieve as low a value for unsharpness as possible, a number of compromises must inevitably be made.

VIEWING THE IMAGE

Much has been said about quantitative evaluation of the performance of the imaging system, but so far little has been said about the performance of the person who uses the image to make a diagnosis.

Performance of the eye

The main factors affecting the performance of the eye are as follows:

- Spectral sensitivity
- Visual acuity
- Recognition acuity
- Detection acuity.

Spectral sensitivity

The spectral sensitivity of the human eye is shown in Figure 9.14. However, this sensitivity depends on whether rod or cone vision is predominant and therefore also depends on the degree of illumination. With cone vision in low levels of illumination

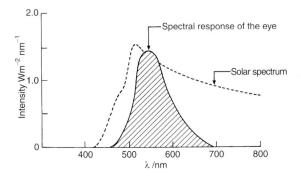

Fig. 9.14 Spectral sensitivity of the human eye.

(e.g. twilight), the peak sensitivity is shifted towards the blue part of the spectrum at 500–560 nm, whereas at high illumination levels (e.g. a sunny day), it is shifted towards the yellow part of the spectrum. Rod vision comes into its own only at very low levels of light intensity (e.g. starlit night). Taken together, this gives the eye a dynamic range in terms of illuminance of about 10 to the power 11.

Visual acuity

Visual acuity can be defined as the ability to perceive spatial detail. It depends on visual angle, luminance and contrast. Figure 9.15 illustrates visual angle (α). It is not the distance of an object that governs whether it will be seen, but the angle that the object subtends to the eye that is important. If the angle exceeds some critical value, the object will be seen. Luminance and contrast are also important factors. The object in Figure 9.15 would be considerably more difficult to see at twilight than in bright sunlight. Likewise, if the object was a snowball in a snow-field it would be impossible to see, as a result of the lack of contrast. The equation of visual angle,

luminance and contrast poses an almost infinite number of variables that prove impossible to simulate in experiments.

Sources suggest that with a 4 mm diameter pupil and a light source of 560 nm, the eye's resolution at 600 mm distance would be approximately 3 lp mm^{-1}. This resolution would alter with distance, and with the use of a magnifying glass. Ideally, if all the cones and rods were evenly distributed across the retina, the eye would have a resolution of 10 000 × 10 000 pixels. Compare this theoretical resolution with a high resolution monitor. It has been suggested that the eye can resolve significantly better than the 3 lp mm^{-1}.

Recognition acuity

This is the ability to recognise a series of standard characters such as letters or specific shapes. Previous experience of the observer can play a significant part in recognition acuity, as practice reduces the time required to spot a particular shape.

Detection acuity

Detection acuity is the ability to detect the presence of an object. Experiments in this area are restricted to detecting simple objects of easily specified structure, as real situations are too complex to model (see Receiver operating characteristics, p. 184). Detection acuity depends on visual angle, contrast and luminance. For example, large objects with low contrast can be seen easily in high levels of illumination. As the object gets smaller and the luminance decreases, the contrast must increase if the object is to remain visible. This leads to the conclusion that in order for an object to be perceived it must exceed some 'perception threshold' that depends on visual

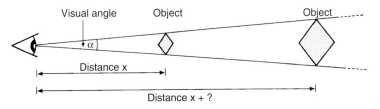

Fig. 9.15 The principle of visual angle. Providing the object at the greater distance subtends the same angle (α) and α is greater than α_{min} then the object will be visualised. It is independent of distance.

angle, contrast and luminance. This threshold must vary from individual to individual, as it depends on the observer's own physiology.

Viewing box

The viewing box must provide an even illumination of the correct colour temperature so that the film being viewed is provided with the best conditions to ensure the highest perceptibility. The light source should be of the northern or tropical daylight type, with a colour temperature of 6500 K. This provides an intense blue/white light which is particularly suitable for use with blue base films. Balance of the intensity of the viewing box light to the ambient room light can significantly improve image quality (see Ch. 10, Quality assurance for exact values in this area, and below, Ambient light, for problems that may arise).

Ambient light

Over recent years, arguments have been presented saying that viewing conditions can have an adverse effect on diagnosis.

In 1981, Dr Bollen, from the Agfa-Gevaert Research Department, presented a paper in San Francisco on this very problem. The paper offers mathematical and visual proof that there is indeed a very serious effect caused by high ambient light: the following explanation is offered:

Behind the patient, the emergent beam will vary between very high and very low levels of intensity. The logarithmic value of these differences can be called the total radiation intensity range (TRIR).

The aim of the recording system is to convert the TRIR into a range of densities. The exposure levels are a product of intensity and time.

Bollen (1981) suggested that three 'phenomena' can be recognised as interfering with perception:

1. The noise of the human visual system, due to the limited number of light photons in the visual detection system at low light levels

2. Dazzling of the observer by extraneous light

3. Visual sensitometric properties caused by reflection on the film surface.

When using a conventional densitometer the light falls specularly on the film.

The 'proper' density is arrived at by measuring the transmitted light (It) and comparing it with the incident light (Io). From this we derive:

$$\text{'Proper' density} = \log \text{Io/It}$$

If an observer views a radiograph, the densities recorded by the eye are correct only if:

1. The spectral sensitivity of the human eye is equal to that of the densitometer

2. The spectral emissions of both light sources are equal

3. There is *no* ambient light

4. Only that particular area is visible to the observer.

If, however, ambient light of intensity Ia falls on the radiograph, part of the light will be reflected back into the observer's eye. This is denoted as Ir.

The 'visual density' will be less than the 'proper density' owing to reflection of the ambient light at the film's surface. If ambient light levels are zero, Ir is equal to 0 and there is no lowering of visual density. However, the following list of figures will give some guide as to the drop which can occur:

$$\text{Ir/It} = \quad 0.5, \text{ density drop} = 0.2$$
$$\text{Ir/It} = \quad 1.0, \text{ density drop} = 0.3$$
$$\text{Ir/It} = \quad 5.0, \text{ density drop} = 0.6$$
$$\text{Ir/It} = 10.0, \text{ density drop} = 1.1$$

In order to test this theoretical approach, Dr Bollen carried out the following experiment. The apparatus used was a Gamma Scientific Spotmeter, which is a telescopic photometer. This was used to measure the visual densities. A Macbeth densitometer was used to measure the proper densities. Both instruments were equipped with an optical filter to match the spectral sensitivity of the eye.

A masked density step wedge was mounted on a viewing box. Using the photometer, light coming from an area of 3 mm^2 was measured at a distance of 1 m. The intensity of the viewing box (Io) was kept at 1700 lux. The ambient light level (Ia) was varied by a dimmer attached to the room lights. Io and Ia were measured by a conventional light photometer.

A number of film types were tested, ranging from grey-dyed gelatine film through conventional black and white films to Medichrome.

It is interesting to note that the black and white films, though of different types and containing different sizes of silver particles, behaved identically. The grey-dyed gelatine film followed the same law as silver bromide films. Some anomalies were found with Medichrome which were mainly due to the differences in colour temperature of the viewing box and the Macbeth light source.

The predicted results, calculated theoretically, coincided almost exactly with the results achieved experimentally. It was discovered that all the films seemed to have a total reflectance of the order of 5–7%. In fact, it meant that 'proper' densities could be converted to 'visual' densities without any need for the telescopic apparatus.

Taking a standard film, the following changes in average gradient were noted:

> 0.0 lux, Average gradient = 3.12
> 50.0 lux, Average gradient = 3.06
> 100.0 lux, Average gradient = 2.94
> 200.0 lux, Average gradient = 2.78
> 500.0 lux, Average gradient = 2.59

It should be stressed that these figures were obtained using net density (ND) 0.25 and ND 1.5, as ND 2.0 was barely achieved at the higher ambient light levels.

In addition to these drops in 'visual' contrast, dramatic losses were noted in the perceptible radiation intensity levels (i.e. perceptibility was drastically reduced).

Perceptibility

It is appreciated that there are essentially three major influences on image quality. They are:

- Contrast
- Unsharpness
- Graininess (noise).

Each of these factors has been explained independently, but it is now time to add all of the information together to produce a common denominator. This is possible because we can reduce the influence of graininess and unsharpness to compensate for changes in contrast. The human eye is capable of perceiving low contrast, but if contrast falls below a certain value the image structure is totally invisible. This value is called the 'contrast threshold' or sometimes the 'minimum contrast'.

A number of other factors also play a part, namely:

- Luminance of the image detail
- Accommodation of the eye
- Glare from the side
- Reflected glare.

As soon as the contrast of the image reaches, or passes, contrast threshold, then in theory the image is clearly seen. This is perceptibility. A knowledge of various contrast thresholds has a great deal of relevance, as perceptibility can be derived for all parts of the radiographic image.

We can say simply that an image structure can be perceived when:

Contrast is equal to, or greater than, the contrast threshold.

If the value of contrast is significantly greater than contrast threshold, then the image structure is easily seen.

Perception, in this context, can be defined as:

The act of discerning the details on the radiograph.

The more the contrast of the image structures exceeds contrast threshold, the higher is the speed of perception.

If the topic of subject contrast is referred to in Chapter 8, Sensitometry, it should be clear that the *subject contrast* must remain within the *film latitude* to give the best potential for the contrast threshold to be exceeded. If it is not within this range (i.e. in the toe or the shoulder of the curve), the potential for reaching contrast threshold is never realised, simply because there is no amplification of subject contrast by the film.

A perceptibility curve

A perceptibility curve provides quantitative data about real system performance by using a suitably designed phantom. From the phantom a number of observers can determine the minimum perceptible radiation contrast at a number of different exposure levels. Average values of all observers are calculated and a graph is plotted using minimum perceptible radiation contrast – $(\Delta \log E)_{min}$ against log E.

Figure 9.16 is an example of such a graph.

Mathematically, it is the distribution function of the number of just perceptible steps. The area under the curve is a measure of the perceptibility. Other graphic measures have also been suggested, such as a plot of minimum perceptible density difference (ΔD_{min}), versus density (Kanomori 1966).

SUMMARY

The perceptibility curve derived for a film will depend upon a number of factors, some of which are listed below:

1. The characteristics of the *observer*

2. The luminance of the *viewing box*

3. The *reflected light* and *glare* conditions

4. *Graininess* can affect the level of the contrast thresholds

5. The *effects of graininess* in general radiography are slight

6. *Unsharpness* can be interpreted, with the help of an *MTF curve*, as a change in detail contrast

7. It is possible to *manipulate the contrast* threshold by altering the contrast factor of

the film, or by dropping the kV. This is only possible if the drop in contrast is *not* due to unsharpness.

A perceptibility curve can completely define image quality, as it takes into account all the parameters which influence diagnosis.

RECEIVER OPERATING CHARACTERISTICS (ROC)

One method of assessing total image quality has been discussed in considering perceptibility, above. Other methods are available but many, while giving values for system or part system performance, ignore the final link in the chain of 'image production', that of the observer who views the radiograph and makes the final diagnosis. It is essential therefore that some system is developed to evaluate the performance of both the system and the observer, to enable a more rational decision to be made on what system suits which observer, and if any particular system consistently gives better results, no matter who observes it.

Principles of receiver operating characteristics

ROC is based on signal detection theory. It is a method of quantifying the ability of an observer to make a diagnosis based on the detection and recognition of, or failure to detect and recognise, some feature in the radiographic image. In the language of *signal detection theory* (SDT), the observer makes a decision as to the existence of a signal in the presence of noise. The decision the observer makes falls into one of four categories:

1. *False positive* (FP). The observer thinks the signal is there when it is not really there (i.e. the observer thinks he/she can see something).

2. *True positive* (TP). The observer thinks the signal is there and it really is there.

3. *True negative* (TN). The observer thinks the signal is not there and it is really not there.

4. *False negative* (FN). The observer thinks the signal is not there when it really is there.

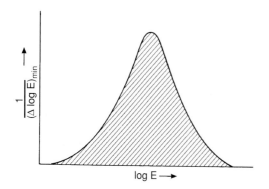

Fig. 9.16 Perceptibility curve.

These four categories are summaries of how the brain's decision mechanism works; the brain, when confronted with a stimulus that it knows may be noise only or signal + noise, has to decide whether the stimulus contains the real signal. When the difference between the signal and noise is large the brain makes few mistakes. However, when it is small and at the threshold of perception, many mistakes may occur. The second case is the most important (e.g. in the early stages of calcification in, say, the breast) and to this end it is in this area (i.e. at the threshold of perception) that SDT experiments are carried out.

Problems in signal detection theory (SDT)

There are many problems in setting up SDT experiments, a few of which are outlined below:

1. Difficulty in simulating the real situation.

2. It is not possible to use real radiographs as they are too complex an item regarding signal and noise (thousands of signal to noise ratios exist on the radiograph). In addition, it must be known which radiographs contains noise only or signal + noise.

3. The observer's previous experience of recognition and classification of the object used (i.e. the signal) significantly improves the results obtained. Not surprisingly, more practice = better results.

4. Time to view each radiograph. If given sufficient time, there is little difficulty in detecting the signal. To eliminate this, a limited viewing time is set.

In order to overcome some of the difficulties, a simplified situation must be created that can be controlled, measured and any conclusions transferred to the real situation.

The simplified situation

In SDT experiments associated with ROC and radiography a situation is created where noise (quantum mottle) varies randomly while the signal (the image of a plastic bead) does not change.

The observer being tested is given a number of radiographs, 50% containing noise only, 50% containing the signal + the noise. The signal to noise ratio varies from film to film, so that in some cases the object is easily seen while in others it is at the perception threshold (i.e. the object can look like noise and the noise can look like the object).

The brain now has to make a decision – 'is there an image there or not?' – for each film. Whenever the signal strength reaching the brain exceeds some critical value (Cv), the brain decides there is an object present. When below Cv the brain responds 'object (signal) not present'. This critical value varies from observer to observer and determines how many mistakes the observer makes.

The decisions the brain can make have been discussed earlier, and are summarised in Figure 9.17.

It is important to note that a large Cv (strict criterion level, as in a careful observer) reduces the number of FP responses but also reduces the TP responses. A low Cv (a lax observer) will correctly pick out nearly all the TP responses but will also make large numbers of FP responses. It has been shown that a person's Cv level varies throughout the day, according to work load, viewing conditions, etc.

The number of responses in each class is recorded and calculated to give:

1. P(S/s) = Probability that a positive response is obtained when there is a signal.

   Therefore: P(S/s) = TP/TP + FN

2. P(S/n) = Probability that a positive response is obtained when there is only noise.

Fig. 9.17 Summary of ROC possible decisions.

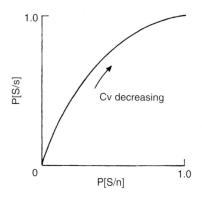

Fig. 9.18 Typical ROC curve.

Therefore: P(S/n) = FP/FP + TN

A graph is now plotted of P(S/s) vs P(S/n): this represents the ROC curve as Cv varies. One observer with a fixed Cv gives one value of P(S/s) and P(S/n) and one point on the graph. Several observers, or criterion levels of Cv, are needed to produce a curve. An example of a curve is shown in Figure 9.18.

Practical procedures of ROC analysis

Procedure 1

The test procedure is the same as in 'The simplified situation' (described above), using 200 radiographs, with 50% noise only and 50% signal plus noise. A single observer views each film in normal viewing conditions. The results are recorded on a separate card for each radiograph, which is numbered to correspond to the number on the film. Observers record on the card, by means of a cross or circle, where they think they see the object on the radiograph. Several observers perform the test and a curve is drawn as previously described. It is important for each observer to keep his/her criterion level (i.e. Cv) the same throughout the experiment.

Procedure 2

This is probably the best method as it allows a curve to be drawn for a single person or group of people.

The test is carried out as before except that the observer is required to make a decision as to the degree of confidence he/she has about his/her response according to the following list:

> 5 = completely confident object present
> 4 = probably present
> 3 = don't know
> 2 = probably not present
> 1 = definitely not present.

This provides each observer with five different criteria levels, enabling a personalised ROC to be drawn.

Tables 9.3 and 9.4 are examples of how the rating procedure is carried out. This in turn can produce a table of values for P(S/s) + P(S/n) (Table 9.5). The ROC curve is now constructed plotting

Table 9.3 ROC results	Category				
	1	2	3	4	5
Number of signal films in category	3	12	35	35	15
Number of noise only films in category	15	35	35	12	3

Table 9.4 ROC results	Categories				
	1 + 2 + 3 + 4 + 5	2 + 3 + 4 + 5	3 + 4 + 5	4 + 5	5
Number of signal films in category	100	97	85	50	
Number of noise only films in category	100	85	50	15	3

Table 9.5	ROC results				
	Category				
	1	2	3	4	5
P (S/s)	1	0.97	0.85	0.50	0.15
P (S/n)	1	0.85	0.50	0.15	0.03

P(S/s) vs P(S/n); this is shown diagrammatically in Figure 9.19.

Interpretation of results

The closer the curve approximates to a right angle, the better the system. This is easily seen by studying Figure 9.20.

As the graph moves from right to left and upwards, the chance of making a positive response when there is a signal is increasing, and the chance of making a positive response when there is only noise, is decreasing; therefore, as previously stated, the closer to a right angle the graph is, the better.

Various ways of quantifying this 'right-angledness' have been proposed, with no firm conclusions to date.

General comment

The preparation of radiographs for this procedure is not a complex process.

Finally, it is important to note that the ROC curves are not confined to one particular situation of, say, low contrast sharp bordered particles but can be drawn for numerous other situations, such as high contrast 'fuzzy'-edged strand objects. ROC curves are very versatile and can assess a system and an observer in almost any situation.

An experiment in ROC analysis

Normal ROC experiments involve the use of one set of radiographs being seen by one observer. This is a time-consuming and laborious process. However, a technique for demonstrating the principles and problems of setting up and taking part in such an experiment has been developed by Dr J. Gore, formerly of the Medical Physics Department of the Hammersmith Hospital. Dr Gore's technique enables quite a large audience to participate in a useful experiment.

The experiment produces a large number of decision matrices at one time, but it is not strictly valid for a number of reasons.

A large number of specimen radiographs with noise and signal + noise are made, and then either mounted directly onto a large format slide carrier or (more practically) copied onto standard 35 mm film.

The resulting slide is projected onto a white screen from several feet (to suit the projection conditions) and viewed by the audience in as dark a condition as is practical. Each participant in the test is asked to decide if the slide being viewed is noise only or signal plus noise, to record this and

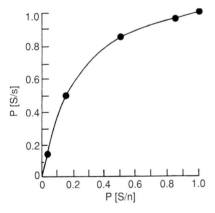

Fig. 9.19 An actual ROC curve (data from Tables 9.3, 9.4 and 9.5).

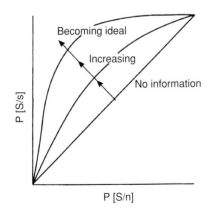

Fig. 9.20 ROC curve – interpretation of results.

to indicate where he/she thinks the signal is (if any) on a card with the slide number.

The observer is told that the signal is a round object and that there may be up to three signals in any one film. The time allowed to view each slide is kept constant at approximately 8–10 seconds.

In order that each participant may produce his/her own personalised ROC and to give the experiment a greater range of results, the observer, as well as indicating the position of the signal, can be asked to show how confident he/she is that the signal is or is not there, using the 1–5 scale outlined in procedure 2, above.

A few of the problems of this experiment are listed below:

- When using the 35 mm format, the ROC is a function not only of the radiographic system but also of the projector system used

- The nature of the viewing screen material: 'daylight' screens tend to increase the noise level

- The angle of view of the observer

- Distance of the observer from the screen

- Degree of background lighting

- Production of results for a group of people

- The fact that the observers know that there are no more than three signals on any one film.

Some advantages of the technique are:

- Allows a large number of participants

- Demonstrates how fatiguing the experiments are to take part in

- Easy to demonstrate the effect of adding or taking away noise or signal by use of a second projector

- Easy to demonstrate effect of change in contrast

- Easy to demonstrate effect of change in object size.

The method used for recording the observers' responses to the test depends on which test is being performed, and can range from a simple 'signal present or not present, delete one not appropriate' to the more popular 'position and certainty' sheet.

REFERENCES

Bollen R 1981 The influence of ambient light. Proceedings of the S.P.I.E. Conference (Medicine), San Francisco 3:22–24

Kanomori H 1966 Determination of optimum film density range for roentgenograms from visual effects. Acta Radiologica 4: 463

Chapter 10
Quality assurance and tests

INTRODUCTION

In radiography, quality assurance is a routine which provides a means of producing high quality radiographs on a day-to-day basis and involves a variety of control procedures being undertaken.

The World Health Organization has defined quality assurance in X-ray medical diagnosis as:

An organised effort by the staff operating a facility to ensure that the diagnostic images produced by the facility are of sufficiently high quality so that they consistently provide adequate diagnostic information at the lowest possible cost and with the least exposure of the patient to radiation.

The objective of a quality assurance programme in an imaging department is to monitor the performance of all the factors which could influence the quality of the image and to try to reduce any film wastage within that department.

In a variety of studies that have been prepared on film wastage, it is often suggested that in some departments wastage can be as high as 20%. In any department, this represents a significant sum of money. Allowances must be made for teaching departments where, of necessity, there must be a higher rejection rate of films. However, an average wastage figure would be of the order of 12% in a department with no form of quality assurance.

If a quality assurance programme is designed for an imaging department it should ideally fulfil the following four main criteria:

1. It should be quantitative, so that repeatability of results is assured
2. It should be simple
3. It should be inexpensive
4. It should be quick.

In a quality assurance programme, it is important that, for example, the results achieved in January can be reproduced the following November.

REJECT ANALYSIS

Preparatory to starting quality assurance in a department, it is wise to do a pilot study of reject (or repeat) analysis of film wastage – i.e. why were films repeated? – to try to establish the norm for the department. The longer the period for these analyses, the better the statistical values obtained.

Method

Stage one

The initial preparation for reject analysis must be to inform *all* the staff that the survey is starting. It is vitally important that all the staff appreciate that cooperation from everyone is essential, otherwise reject analysis will become meaningless.

The aims of the project should be stressed:

- To try to identify where, and why, the wastage is occurring
- To try to reduce the overall costs within the imaging department.

It is also very important for the staff to appreciate that the analysis is not a 'witch hunt' with the aim of identifying poor radiographers, but is merely an assessment of the current conditions.

Stage two

A period of 8–10 weeks is set aside to conduct the survey, ideally starting on a Monday morning and finishing on a Friday night.

Before the Monday morning start, *all* film in the department must be identified, counted and the *details recorded*.

The easiest way of achieving this is to empty all cassettes, the film hopper and any partially empty boxes. This film is then set aside until the end of the survey, when it can be used again.

To ensure accuracy of the records, a check must then be kept, on a daily basis, of all films removed from the film stores.

Stage three

It is advised that all film analysis should be conducted on a daily basis. The volume of films which may be rejected, and then have to be sorted, should deter anyone from attempting to do a weekly check.

The rejected films should then be sorted out into categories. Some suggested categories are listed below:

1. Positioning

2. Movement

3. Too light

4. Too dark (unknown whether films are over- or underexposed: may be machine/processor/screen problem)

5. Processing (marks, scratches, etc.)

6. Others (screen artefacts, light beam diaphragms, etc.)

7. Rejects by room.

The categories listed are not the only ones that can be used, of course. For example, it would be possible to identify the cassettes used for the rejected films.

There is a lot of information to be gained from a survey such as this and the statistical evidence produced can be interpreted and used in many ways.

Information can be gained about particular rooms which may be consistently faulty. Cassettes and screens may be identified which are outside speed tolerances. Persistent faults in a room may point to a misunderstanding of the equipment, perhaps even to more 'in-house training', for example. The survey may not just prove how costly the department is to run. It can also be used to justify extra staff, for example, if records can prove this need.

Analysis

At the end of the period, all films remaining in the department must be counted. The films used will be known, because of the record of movement of film from the film store. The total number of films used can now be obtained.

If possible, weekly analyses should be obtained of film usage. This will give an even better statistical evaluation.

Figures 10.1 and 10.2 indicate just one way in which the statistics obtained from a reject analysis survey may be presented. The figures

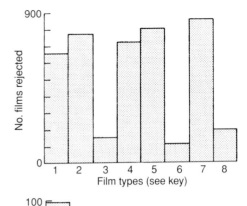

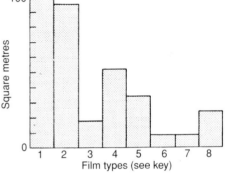

Key to the histograms.

Size	Number of films	Square metres
1. 35 × 43	660	99.33
2. 35 × 35	777	95.18
3. 30 × 40	153	18.36
4. 24 × 40	727	52.34
5. 18 × 24	807	34.86
6. 18 × 43	113	8.75
7. 100 mm	863	8.63
8. Other*	200	24.06
Total	4300	341.51

* CT, duplicating film, copy films, occlusals, etc.

Figs. 10.1 and 10.2 Presentation of statistics obtained from a reject analysis survey.

obtained are from an actual survey conducted in a large imaging department.

Many books advise that the analysis is produced by taking the percentage of *films* rejected. While this is adequate, there is a major flaw in this argument (which is illustrated in the figures). If the aim is to assess the wastage of film, the best guide is to find the total *square metreage* rejected. This final figure will give a very good guide to the actual cost: 20, 18 × 24s do not represent the same cost as 20, 35 × 43s!

Table 10.1 shows the square metreage of film in boxes of 100 films.

It is only reasonable to point out that the percentage figures arrived at do not always tell the whole story. It is suggested that reject analysis does not take into account two important factors: diagnostic criteria and compensation.

Diagnostic criteria

In this case the radiologist accepts a film for diagnosis, even though it would normally be unacceptable, because it would be very difficult or impossible to repeat it.

The problem outlined in 'diagnostic criteria' is a root problem unique to medical radiography. It effectively means that there is no 'standard' radiograph for each examination.

Compensation

In this case the radiographer makes allowances for a room which is known to take 'the extra 5 kV', or a faulty cassette which needs a 'little bit more'. In other words the radiographer compensates for an already known fault.

Having established the percentage rejection/square metreage rate, other factors in the department must be investigated. This will then lead to a complete quality assurance programme.

THE QUALITY ASSURANCE PROGRAMME

AREAS TO MONITOR

There are four main areas which need to be monitored closely if quality assurance is to be undertaken. They are as follows:

Image producers

- X-ray set
- Associated chain of equipment
- Could include the image intensifier, etc.

Image receptors

- X-ray intensifying screens
- X-ray film
- Television monitors could also be included.

Image processors

- Processing machine found in the imaging department.

Viewing system

- Conventional viewing boxes.

APPARATUS REQUIRED

The following list represents a minimum requirement for apparatus if a quality assurance programme is to be undertaken in the department:

- Densitometer
- Contact test grid
- An ultraviolet light, the output to be 250 nm or below
- A calibrated step wedge, *or* a sensitometer, *or* manufacturer's pre-exposed step wedge film
- An alcohol thermometer, plus a maximum–minimum thermometer
- A hydrometer

Table 10.1 Square metreage per box of 100 films	
Film size × 100	Square metres
13 × 18 cm	= 2.34
15 × 40 cm	= 6.00
18 × 24 cm	= 4.32
20 × 40 cm	= 8.00
24 × 30 cm	= 7.20
30 × 40 cm	= 12.00
35 × 35 cm	= 12.25
35 × 43 cm	= 15.05
$6\frac{1}{2} \times 8\frac{1}{2}$ in	= 3.56
8 × 10 in	= 5.16
10 × 12 in	= 7.75
12 × 15 in	= 11.62
7 × 17 in	= 7.74
15 × 6 in	= 5.79

- A pH meter, relative humidity meter, silver estimating papers; light meter.

To give some idea of the preparations involved in the setting up of a quality assurance programme, the document issued by Agfa-Gevaert preparatory to starting the programme is set out below. Each section of the programme is dealt with in much greater detail later in the chapter.

Setting up a quality assurance programme (extracted from the Agfa-Gevaert Diagnostic Imaging Systems Division document)

On the first day, the major processor in the department will be needed to find the optimum temperature for this processor. This is a time-consuming exercise and the processor will most probably be required for the whole day. *It should not be switched on for this morning.*

Following this evaluation, an X-ray room will be required to complete the cassette/screen evaluation. This room *must* produce consistent reproducible exposures, otherwise the tests will be invalid. This can only be assessed by testing. The length of time taken for the cassette/screen survey is dependent on the number of cassettes to be surveyed. As a guide, a full survey of 150 cassettes will require about 4 working days.

The rest of the survey will be conducted around the work of the department.

A full report will be produced at the end of the quality assurance evaluation.

Note: It is not considered that X-ray machine evaluation is part of the responsibility of a film manufacturer. However, if faults are suspected, this information will be communicated to the department head for further action.

IMAGE PROCESSORS

It is perhaps wisest to consider first the apparatus which processes the image, the automatic processor.

The automatic processor is an essential piece of apparatus in virtually every imaging department, and almost every film produced passes through it.

In the days of totally manual processing, there was a great deal of flexibility in the procedure, and temperature or time could be adjusted to accommodate variations in processing solutions. Not so with an automatic processor. Time, temperature and replenishment are closely controlled.

Even very large imaging departments may have only two processors, so any faults which develop can affect a large number of films over a fairly short time.

So much of quality assurance is the practical application of the knowledge of photochemistry and sensitometry in addition to the basic understanding of screens and phosphors.

PROCESSOR EVALUATION

The objective of these tests is:

- To ensure that the processor is operating at peak performance and optimum temperature

- To identify any possible problems, so that any corrective action may be taken to ensure that the processor remains at peak performance.

Test equipment

Electric pH meter

This meter is calibrated on site to standard solutions. Its primary use is to establish accurate pH readings and thereby to ensure correct replenishment rates.

Silver estimating papers

When these papers are immersed in fixer they change colour. This colour change is matched against a colour chart. This match gives an indication of the quantity of silver in the fixer in grams per litre (g/l). Too high a silver level can be caused by under-replenishment or blockage and will certainly result in incomplete fixing of the film.

Residual thiosulphate test solution

When a drop of this solution is placed on each side of the film, a stain appears. The shade of this stain is matched to a colour chart to indicate whether all the residual chemicals have been washed from the emulsion. This gives an indication of the archival life of the film, which certainly should be in excess of 10 years.

Alcohol thermometer

Used for direct measurements of solution temperatures. A mercury thermometer is *not* recommended in a photographic area as accidental breakages can cause numerous photographic faults.

Sensitometer

The sensitometer used is calibrated to a standard wedge. The unit is capable of producing a green light emission, suitable for orthochromatic films, as well as a blue light source.

The sensitometric strip produced is a 21 step wedge, also known as a 'root 2' wedge. This image is particularly suitable for quality assurance, as it offers a detailed 21 step wedge for accuracy, but for regular use it can be used for a three step system.

Densitometer

Densitometers automatically read the relative density of the various steps on the film by measuring the quantity of light which passes through an area. The more light that passes through, the lower the density. This information can either be directly read off the LED display for each step and then the characteristic curve plotted by hand, or, in the more sophisticated models, the densitometer can be linked to a computer and all the steps are automatically read. The quality control information can then be automatically printed along with the characteristic curve for the film. In addition, information can be stored and weekly or monthly print-outs produced, if required, to show the trends in processor activity and to allow comparisons between various processors that the department may have.

PROCESSOR CHECKS

As well as checking the purely mechanical side of the operation of the processor, there are chem-ical checks which must be done to ensure the smooth running of the unit.

After considering what are basically mechanical checks on agitation, temperature, speed and replenishment, the chemical and sensitometric performance of the processor must be checked by monitoring the following:

- *Developer*, in terms of pH variations and sensitometric performance. Specific gravity measurements should also be considered.

- *Fixer*, in terms of pH variations and silver levels within the fixer. Specific gravity measurements should also be considered.

Mechanical checks

The suppliers of the automatic processor will have literature available which will advise on how to carry out routine mechanical inspections. It is very important to note replenishment rates and to know how to correct them. While no piece of mechanical apparatus can be considered to be perfect, the modern automatic processor is basically a very reliable unit.

With the advent of area scanning of film, replenishment rates have become very accurate as now the *area* of the film is measured, rather than only the *length*.

Chemical checks

pH

Each chemical manufacturer supplies details of the pH operating levels of the developer and fixer. An electric pH meter is the most suitable way of obtaining accurate pH measurements. Automatic processing developers, with few exceptions, range between 9.0 and 10.6, while automatic fixers range between 4.0 and 5.0. Ideally pH should be measured daily, although many departments carry out weekly measurements, measuring replenishment rates at the same time.

No matter how often measurements are made, it is most important to record the measurements. Many people consider that as the measurements are always the same, it seems unnecessary to check them and even more unnecessary to record them.

The routine measurement of pH is not a very time-consuming task, but if it is logged regularly it can provide some very important information. In the graphs of pH the following parameters apply.

1. The developer pH is assumed to be a norm of 10.00 in the machine tank and the replenisher pH is 10.3.

2. The fixer pH is assumed to be 4.4 in the machine and replenisher tanks.

3. It is assumed that daily measurements are made.

Figure 10.3 illustrates what would happen when there is gross over-replenishment of developer over a period of days. There is a gradual increase of pH, due to the fact that the replenisher has a higher pH than the machine tank developer. Gradually, the basic fog will begin to rise, as the machine tank developer is now becoming unselective due to its increased activity. The rise in basic fog will cause a fall in average gradient as the slope of the curve will be altered.

Gross under-replenishment causes the pH to drop (Fig. 10.4). This produces a fall in average gradient, now due to the fact that the developer is not as active (low pH), so maximum densities are not reached on the film. The change in the slope of the curve also gives an apparent decrease in the film's speed.

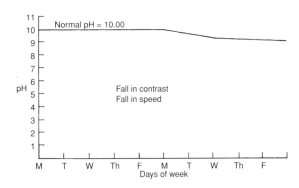

Fig. 10.4 Developer grossly under-replenished.

When fixer pH is measured with gross over-replenishment, there is no discernible effect. However, with gross under-replenishment (Fig. 10.5), many problems can be caused. The pH now increases, owing to carry-over of the developer which cannot be buffered by an under-replenished fixer. The higher the pH, the worse the problems become, but they are typically:

• *Transport problems* due to the film swelling excessively in the wash water because of inadequate hardening

• *Scratches* due to a very soft non-hardened emulsion

• *Non-drying* because of excess water in the emulsion

• At the very worst, a fall in average gradient due to a *milky white overall fog* shown on the film due to non-fixation.

The following has been mentioned before, but no apologies are included for mentioning it

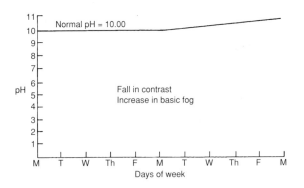

Fig. 10.3 Developer grossly over-replenished.

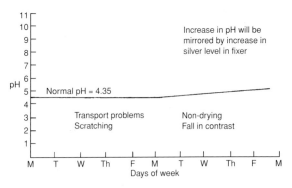

Fig. 10.5 Fixer grossly under-replenished.

again. Many people assume that, because results do not vary, the quality assurance system is not working. The whole point of quality assurance is that the measurements *should* always be the same. The results *should* always be negative. The aim of these measurements is to spot a trend and, if necessary, stop it.

Specific gravity

The measurement of specific gravity can be very useful if there are any doubts about too much, or too little, water being added to a mix. Again, manufacturers will supply details of the specific gravity of their chemicals.

If the measured specific gravity is too low, then the solutions are too dilute (i.e. somehow too much water has been added). If the specific gravity is too high, not enough water has been added.

Be aware of one major trap if specific gravity has to be measured. All hydrometers are calibrated according to temperature. If the hydrometer is calibrated at 20°C then the liquid must be brought to that temperature before making the measurement.

More information on the behaviour of developer and fixer is contained in Chapter 6, Photochemistry.

Fixer silver level

The most accurate way of checking that the fixer is being replenished correctly is to measure the silver content of the fixer. This can be done very quickly and easily using silver estimating papers.

These are dipped into the fixer tank, and the colour change is compared to a colour chart supplied with the papers. For a 90 s processor the level should be about 6–7 g of silver per litre of fixer. A typical processor will contain about 120–140 g of silver, which is all recoverable. The user should be aware that these papers are called silver *estimating* papers and only provide a guide to the silver content. The papers should be renewed regularly; about once a year is sufficient.

Sensitometric checks

The automatic processor should process a film correctly. This seems a trite statement, but the only way to find whether this is happening is to do some form of sensitometric check and compare the results with the manufacturer's published figures.

The performance of the film in the automatic processor should be maximised. This can be done fairly simply, although the tests themselves are very time-consuming unless computer software is available to speed up the process.

Fog, speed, average gradient

The automatic processor should be started from cold and then a series of measurements are made at 1°C intervals. The range of temperature measurements will depend on the type of chemistry in use, i.e. whether it is 'cold' or 'hot' developer.

Sensitometric strips are then fed through the machine at the 1°C intervals. Plots are then made of:

- Basic fog versus temperature
- Speed versus temperature
- Average gradient versus temperature.

It can be considered that the chemistry and processor performance will be maximised when the fog is at an acceptable level (i.e. below density 0.22) and the speed is as high as possible when compared to the average gradient. It should be noted that the average gradient will climb gradually and then begin to fall as the basic fog increases. The optimum temperature will be about 1°C below the maximum average gradient achieved, with acceptable fog level (Fig. 10.6).

Once the optimum settings are obtained, a three patch system can be adopted for routine tests. For the simplest method of sensitometry which is still accurate, three areas are required for measurement using a densitometer (Figure 10.7).

These three areas can be considered as the following:

1. *Basic fog.* As measured at patch A.
2. *Speed index.* Value of density at patch B.
3. *Contrast index.* Value of density at patch C.

Note that points 2 and 3 are *indices* and only represent a point on the curve and not an absolute value for speed and contrast.

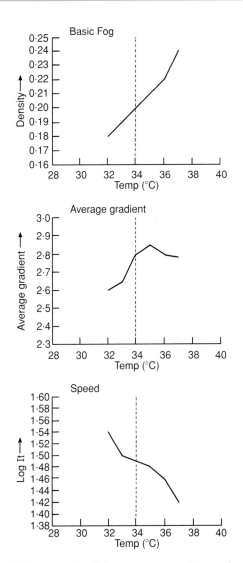

Fig. 10.6 Plots of basic fog, average gradient and speed against temperature.

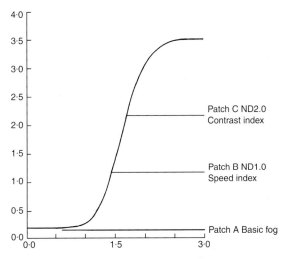

Fig. 10.7 Three patch system: basic fog, speed index and contrast index.

Once the curve is produced on a day-to-day basis, these same three values are always measured and recorded. It is now that trends may be observed (Fig. 10.8).

If the speed index goes up or down, it means that the apparent speed of the film has done the same. If the contrast index goes up or down, so has the average gradient on the film.

Ideally, if the curves are being produced on film from the department, a specific box should be designated for such tests. When the changeover to a new box of film occurs, a film

from the old box and the new box should be exposed together. This precaution is necessary, as there might be a difference in sensitivity between different emulsions. Any difference in densities should be noted and the resultant differences recorded. This slight change is important to note. If, for example, the starting density at B was D1.2, as in the graph, and at changeover the value was D1.3, then this is the *new starting point* for B (Fig. 10.9). Exactly the same rules would apply to patches C and A.

Figure 10.10 shows the changes that can occur using this method. It is important to realise that it is a trend that is being looked for, not a massive sensational swing.

Using a densitometer, the results can easily be achieved and certain defined limits can be made for allowable swings. Variations of D0.15, either up or down, will mean a move which is out of tolerance. Most radiographers find a basic fog much greater than 0.22 unacceptable. The variations allowable for both speed and contrast indices above and below the starting value are D0.15 (Fig. 10.10).

Without a densitometer, some guesswork has to be done, but fairly accurate results can still be obtained. An increase or decrease in basic fog can be estimated, as can the speed index. Unfortunately, because the contrast index is above density 2, it is impossible to

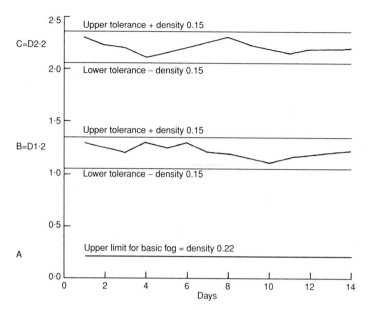

Fig. 10.8 The start at C is the measured density of patch C; the start at B is the measured density at patch B; the value of A is the measured value of basic fog. The maximum and minimum values around these values are shown. The starting density values of all three patches will vary, according to types and batches of films used.

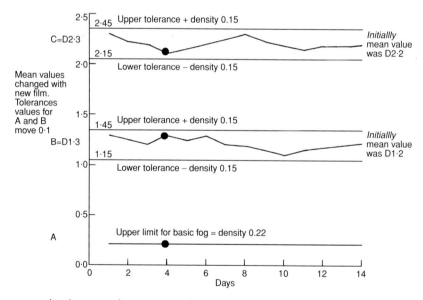

Fig. 10.9 ● represents the change at day 4 to a new batch of film. The old values at A, B and C are changed to the new values on the new film. The only proviso is that an old and new film should be processed together (see text).

make a reliable estimate of increase or decrease in density. Even so, 70% of potential problems can be spotted using purely visual qualitative estimates.

Computerised processor control

Systems are now available which involve computer software to monitor the processing equipment.

Trends exhibited		Possible causes of trends
/	Basic fog	Excess developer in fixer
/	Speed index	Faulty developer preparation
\	Contrast index	Insufficient mixing
/	Basic fog	Insufficient starter added to developer
\	Speed index	Over-replenishment of developer
\	Contrast index	Completely oxidised developer
—	Basic fog	Developer over-diluted
\	Speed index	Under-replenishment of developer
\	Contrast index	
/	Basic fog	Developer temperature too high
/	Speed index	Faulty preparation of developer
/	Contrast index	Insufficient mixing
\	Basic fog	Developer temperature too low
\	Speed index	Exhausted or under-replenished developer
\	Contrast index	Faulty developer preparation
/	Basic fog	Fixer in developer
—	Speed index	Under-replenished fixer
\	Contrast index	

Fig. 10.10   Trends of basic fog, speed index and contrast index, and some possible causes of those trends.

Sensitometric control strips are processed and then the 21 steps are read by passing them through a 'strip reader'. Calculations are then automatically made which determine the speed, contrast and fog level. The information is stored and a characteristic curve is produced and evaluated. The evaluation of the curve may also state whether or not the curve is within normal limits and suggest steps (including other tests) which can be taken to rectify the fault. Normal values are given and several characteristic curves can be displayed together to enable comparisons to be easily and quickly made.

SAFELIGHT EVALUATION

Safelights are a specialised application of optical filters. Their function is to provide a high level of 'darkroom' illumination without any detrimen-

tal effect on the sensitive material (film) that is being handled. They thus provide the darkroom worker with a more acceptable environment than working in complete darkness, although this is still sometimes necessary.

Safelights used in radiographic darkrooms come in two types, but both depend on the same principle of operation.

Principle of operation of safelights

Their basis of operation is the selective optical filtering of a white light source in such a manner that the film material being handled is subject only to wavelengths to which it is not sensitive.

The performance of a particular filter can be assessed by plotting the percentage of light transmitted through the filter at selected wavelengths throughout the visible spectrum; alternatively, due to the relationship between transmittance and density (see Ch. 8, Sensitometry), by plotting filter density at particular wavelengths. Because in practice film sensitivity and safelight performance are linked, it is traditional to superimpose the film spectrogram onto the safelight transmittance properties, as Figure 10.11 illustrates. This allows the user to see at a glance if any wavelength of the light transmitted is close to the spectral sensitivity of the film. The manufacturer will almost always recommend a suitable safelight for a particular film, but generally the following are used:

- For monochromatic emulsions an orange safelight
- For orthochromatic a dark red safelight
- For panchromatic total darkness.

Factors affecting safelight performance

The main factors affecting safelight performance are:

- Distance from the darkroom bench
- Wattage of the bulb
- Number and position of safelights
- Spectral emission features of the filters
- White light leakage
- Safe handling time.

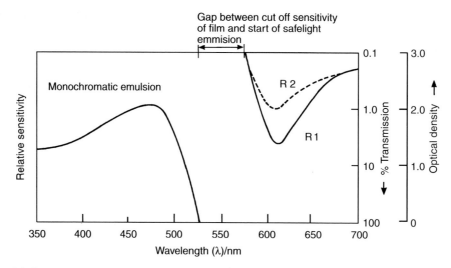

Fig. 10.11 Safelight transmission features versus film spectral sensitivity, showing a 'safe' combination with two different safelight filters: R1 and R2.

Distance and bulb wattage

The recommended distance between the safe-light and the working bench depends principally on the wattage of the bulb in the safelight. The higher the wattage, the further away it needs to be 'safe' (inverse square law applies).

For a direct ('beehive'-type) safelight with a 25 W pearl tungsten filament bulb, the recommended closest distance is 1.2 m; this may be reduced to 0.6 m if a 15 W bulb is used. In an indirect safelight (i.e. one that depends entirely on reflection from the walls and ceiling of the darkroom to provide illumination), bulb wattage may be up to 60 W, but careful testing must be carried out to ensure safety.

Number and position

The number of safelights governs the overall illumination of the darkroom. Darkrooms should not be 'dark'; they should have sufficient 'safe light' to be able to work without undue difficulty, commensurate with keeping the fog level on the film to a minimum. One indirect light for every 6 m² of ceiling area at a height of 2 m above floor level should be sufficient to provide a good general level of illumination. Specific areas of the bench can be specially illuminated by using a 'direct'-type safelight. Too many and/or badly positioned safelights can have a significant effect on the base + fog level of the film, and can therefore influence image quality.

Spectral emission

The specific details are covered in principles of operation (above). However, the problem arises from 'mismatching' the spectral emission of the safelight with the sensitivity of the film, for example an orange safelight with an orthochromatic film emulsion.

White light leakage

A cracked or damaged filter or housing may be leaking minute amounts of white light, totally invisible to the naked eye but easily 'seen' by the film. At low intensity levels this would be more than sufficient to raise the base + fog level to an unacceptable degree.

Safe handling time

This is the length of time the film may be handled in normal safelight conditions without an increase in the base + fog level. In a general darkroom this should be approximately 45 seconds. All the factors listed above can affect this, therefore routine testing of the safe handling time should be undertaken.

The International Organisation for Standardisation (ISO) safelight test

ISO 8374 – Photography – Determination of ISO safelight conditions was first published in December 1986. It contains a full description of the pre-exposure, post-exposure tests and the test used during the processing cycle, along with a glossary of definitions.

This standard is deemed applicable to 'all wet or dry photographic films, plates and papers'. What follows is a practical application of this ISO Standard and many definitions included in the glossary have, of necessity, been excluded. However, the definition of the ISO safelight condition is:

> **Lighting conditions that provide less than one-half the exposure required to produce a photographic effect when evaluated by use of the methods described in the International Standard.**

Test equipment

A pre-exposed step tablet is highly recommended for use in this test, unless direct X-radiation (as opposed to light from intensifying screens) normally produces the image, in which case X-radiation should be used. If a step tablet is not available, the following procedure should be used:

The film is given a flash exposure which will take it past threshold, to a density of about 0.6. This action sensitises the film and reproduces the normal film use. A degree of practice is needed to achieve this result using white light. If necessary, the film can be loaded into a cassette and an exposure of 5 mAs and 40 kV, with a class 100 system will produce satisfactory exposure.

The piece of sensitised material should be covered with two pieces of opaque black card, ensuring that the top 2.5 cm strip of the film remains covered and therefore unexposed. The next 2.5 cm are uncovered in turn as each strip is given an exposure (using a light of the same spectral quality as that of the intensifying screens) using a series of exposure times (e.g. 1 s, 2 s, 4 s, 8 s, 16 s, 32 s, etc.) and using the card to uncover a different strip of film for each exposure. If this film was processed it would have the appearance of a film made by using a step wedge. An accurate timer is also required.

Data recording

A record should be kept of all pertinent data such as:

- Safelight filter designation
- Size
- Age
- Lamp type
- Wattage and voltage
- Distance from filter to film
- Sensitised film type
- Safelight exposure times
- Processing data.

Note must also be taken of the physical condition of the filter material such as fading, cracking, etc.

Once the correct figures have been obtained it is important that the environment is not changed (e.g. painting the darkroom walls, distances from the bench, etc.); finally, the darkroom procedures for film handling and processing should be carefully controlled.

Testing the safelights

The 'step wedge' film is placed on the bench in total darkness. The film should be covered with two pieces of opaque black card ensuring the left (or right!) 2.5 cm strip of the film remains covered and therefore unexposed (this strip will included an image of all the 'steps' of the step wedge and will be used for comparison purposes). The next 2.5 cm are uncovered in turn as each strip is given an exposure to the safelights to be tested using a series of exposure times, each exposure time being increased by a factor of 2 (e.g. 4 s, 8 s, 16 s, 32 s, etc.) and using the card to uncover a different strip of film for each exposure.

The film is processed within 2 hours of exposure (to minimise latent image fade) in the usual processor.

Evaluation

The densities of all the strips are measured. The density of the strips which have been exposed to safelights are compared with the strip which was not exposed to safelights. The strip which received the most safelight exposure without increasing the density of any step is determined. The exposure time of this final strip is then divided by 2, giving the 'ISO safelight condition'.

IMAGE RECEPTORS

This covers three main topics;

- Film
- Intensifying screens
- Cassettes.

X-RAY FILM EVALUATION

Although the performance of the film can be monitored by the consumer, there is very little that can be done about the quality of the film. All film manufacturers have stringent quality assurance procedures which involve detailed batch sampling and close monitoring of production and packing, etc. It would be incorrect to say that film faults are not produced in the manufacturing process, but they are few and far between.

There are, however, two areas where the consumer can take care of the quality of the film *after* it has reached the imaging department.

Stock control

All film has a shelf life. This simply means that the film has a useful life during which it can be expected that it will maintain its manufactured quality. After this period, usually indicated by an expiry date on the box, the quality of the film begins to deteriorate and the overall basic fog will begin to increase. It is therefore essential to make absolutely sure that X-ray film is used in strict rotation.

For example:

1. When films are received into the department they should be date stamped, or identified in some way so that the date of entry into the department is known.

2. They should then be used in strict rotation – for example, First In are First Out, or Last In are Last Out provide two useful mnemonics, FIFO and LILO. If this practice is followed, there should be no possibility of finding 3-year-old boxes of film on the shelf.

Storage conditions

1. Always store film vertically, not horizontally. If films are stored horizontally, it is almost certain that pressure marks will be produced on those at the bottom of the pile.

2. Try to maintain an even temperature in the storage area. An ideal way to check the temperature swings is to use a maximum–minimum thermometer. The swing should be relatively low, perhaps of the order of 1–2°C. The ideal temperature would be 10°C if the films are to be stored for longer than 3 months. Film can be stored in temperatures much lower than this with no detrimental effect. Significantly higher temperatures will only hasten the ageing process.

3. Make sure that the storage area is not damp. For example, hot water pipes passing through a storage room can cause condensation. A value of about 50% relative humidity should be aimed for.

4. Avoid storing photographic chemicals in the same area as the film. Spillage of the chemicals can obviously cause problems. There is an additional hazard as well: a number of developers contain minute quantities of a radioactive isotope of potassium. If films have to be in the same storage area as chemicals, keep the film at least 2 m away from the developer.

5. Certain fumes are known to fog films, carbon monoxide (car exhausts), formalin and formaldehyde (typical laboratory chemicals) and certain types of paint, to name but a few.

6. Mercury vapour will also fog film. *Never* use a mercury thermometer in a photographic dark-

room. If a mercury thermometer is broken inside an automatic processor, the problems are enormous. Mercury 'kills' developer and also forms an amalgam with stainless steel. The processor will require a great deal of cleaning, possibly even a replacement tank.

7. Finally, consider carefully the building materials used in the construction of a film storage area. Avoid materials such as breeze block if possible, as some constituents may well be minutely radioactive.

FILM EVALUATION

Residual thiosulphate test

This assesses the archival permanence of the processed film. It can be carried out using a commercially available preparation,. To carry out the test, place a small drop of the solution on the emulsion surface in a clear area of the film to be tested. If the film is duplitised, this should be in the same place on both emulsions. Blot off the excess using a paper towel and wait the period of time recommended in the instructions (usually about 30 seconds, in subdued lighting). Compare the colour on the film with the comparator chart and assess the archival permanence range. This should be carried out in daylight to obtain the most accurate results. Do not place the film on a viewing box after the solution has been applied, as this accelerates the reaction that is occurring and gives a false indication of the archival permanence; also, do not attempt to compare the film with the colour chart after about 30 seconds beyond the recommended waiting time as this also gives false indications.

If thiosulphate is present, it is indicated by a yellow coloration that gets progressively darker the worse the archival permanence.

INTENSIFYING SCREEN AND CASSETTE EVALUATION

Screens and cassettes are interlinked in such a way that the testing procedures and the quality assurance procedures for both are described

together. Radiographers find it strange, when repeating a 'thin' film, that after giving a reasonable increase in exposure, the new film is grossly overexposed. The X-ray set is blamed, then the processor, even the film itself, but very rarely is the intensifying screen suspected. It is quite possible that the repeat film was done on a different cassette, with screens theoretically the same but in fact with a different age. It is in cases like this that quality assurance comes into its own.

The objectives of the tests are:

1. To determine any loss of film/screen contact
2. To determine the presence of any scratches or abrasion damage to the screen
3. To determine any speed variations due to the age and condition of the screen.

Test equipment

Screen contact tester

A special test tool is required for this procedure which contains a perforated metal sheet. The test tool is laid flat on the face of the cassette and an exposure is made at approximately 55 kV at 2 m focus-film distance, the processed film being viewed at 4 m. If contact is uniform, the film in turn will show overall uniform density. Areas of high density will indicate a loss of screen contact in the area of the dark patches (see p. 205).

Ultraviolet (UV) light

This UV light emits light at a wavelength of 250 nm. This particular wavelength is extremely suitable for activating the screen phosphors. When the screen is scanned with the UV light, the surface phosphors are excited and artefacts and abrasions are readily discerned.

Densitometer

The densitometer used is calibrated on site to a standard step wedge.

Numbering

It is very important to number cassettes, both inside and out. This makes identification of a faulty screen, for example, very easy. Various types of numbers exist commercially to do just this job.

Routine cleaning

1. Always clean screens with the cleaning solution recommended by the manufacturer of the screens. Some screen cleaning solutions from manufacturer A will damage screens made by manufacturer B.

2. Never use soap and water. Even after apparently through washing some soap can be left on the supercoat. Eventually this can discolour, and will then act as a filter for the light emitted by the screen. In addition, accumulated layers of the soap can become radio-absorptive. These two factors, emission down and X-ray reduction, can produce a much slower screen system. Cleaning with water may lead to other problems when dealing with rare earth screens (see p. 84). *All* rare earths are hygroscopic. If the screen supercoat is damaged, water may be absorbed by the phosphor, causing discoloration of the supercoat and therefore a reduction of the light emission and subsequent loss of speed.

3. Normal everyday dust and dirt should be removed with a soft brush, such as a camera lens cleaning brush. For more ingrained dirt, use a lint-free cloth and screen cleaner, rubbing in a circular motion without undue pressure. If a great deal of effort is required to remove the dirt from the screens, it is almost certain that the dirt is already too far embedded into the supercoat of the screen.

4. Once the screens have been cleaned, leave the cassettes partially open so the screens can dry naturally.

The act of using a screen cleaner has two specific benefits. The cleaner obviously cleans the screens, but most screen cleaners contain an anti-static element. A considerable amount of static can be generated simply by the act of inserting and extracting the film from the cassette. Static in turn will attract dirt and dust.

Drying the screens is essential, as some components of screen cleaners, when in contact with film, can fog the emulsion if the screen is still wet.

Inspection

Stage one. After the screens have been cleaned thoroughly, they have to be inspected in white light. If the screens are examined by reflected light, any bad surface marks and scratches will usually show up quite readily. Any screens with marks in the central area should be put to one side for further tests.

Stage two. All X-ray screen phosphors operate by converting short wave energy into long wave, usually visible, energy. If a short wave source can be found that will excite the phosphors, they will fluoresce. An X-ray tube performs this service admirably, but is extremely impractical for prolonged testing. Fortunately, ultraviolet light, with a wavelength of about 250 nm, will also excite X-ray phosphors. The test procedure is as follows.

The cassettes are laid out flat on a darkroom bench and then all the lights in the darkroom are switched off. The intensifying screens are then scanned, using the ultraviolet light source. As the UV light actually makes the phosphor fluoresce, any defect, such as fingermarks or areas of diminished light output, will be clearly seen.

Warning: Prolonged exposure to UV light can cause conjunctivitis. UV light of 250 nm is readily absorbed by the glass in a pair of spectacles and should be safe for most users, but care must be taken.

If any faults are demonstrated on this test, particularly if they lie in the central area of the screens, the screens are moved on to the next test procedure.

Stage three. It is possible that screens were rejected in the first stage; these are collected with the rejected cassettes from the second stage and are now examined using X-radiation. This part of the test increases quite dramatically the cost of a quality assurance programme. It should only be used as a last resort, to confirm that the marks demonstrated visually are confirmed by

X-radiation. It is possible that the cassettes could be passed on to the screen contact test, but sometimes small artefacts are not visible on a screen contact test. Essentially this test should be used with considered judgement.

These cassettes are loaded with film and placed under the X-ray tube. In this instance, distance is not so critical and the tube can be raised to the limits of its vertical travel to provide the largest area coverage possible. A 'flash exposure' is then given, about 10 mAs and 55 kV for 'universal'-type screens, and the films are then processed.

When the films are viewed after processing, any artefacts will be clearly seen as the films will have a density of somewhere around 1.0. It is then that the difficult decision about which cassettes to reject must be made. Obviously any artefact which resembles phleboliths or calculi must be immediately suspected and rejected. The rest of the marks remain with the conscience of the user.

Screen contact

In the inspection stage, it is quite possible that a number of cassettes have been rejected on the basis of unacceptable marks on the screens. The remaining cassettes must now be tested for screen contact. Fortunately, the screen contact test also has an inbuilt test for the speed of the screens.

Reproducibility

Before commencing the test there is one precaution which must be observed. As the screen contact test can also be used as a speed test it is imperative that the X-ray set used for the tests is working correctly. This can be checked by making a number of exposures on one cassette, carefully masking the film for each exposure. When measured with a densitometer each exposure should have produced the same density. A deviation in density of about 5% is acceptable. If the deviations are greater than this, the set is not giving reproducible exposures and another set must be found and the tests done again.

To confirm reproducibility during the tests, one cassette, ideally of a small format, should be chosen as a control cassette. This cassette, loaded with film, should be placed in the centre of every group of cassettes which is exposed during the tests. The same density should be recorded on this control cassette after every exposure.

Problems also occur with the anode heel effect. As a precaution, a record should be kept of the position of every cassette during the tests. If density variations are found from 'north' to 'south', but are similar in all test exposures, the variations can be assumed to be caused by a similar effect.

British Standard tests

The test for screen contact is covered by British Standard BS7725-2.2 1994 and IEC 61223-2-2 1993. These standards cover cassettes, film changers and film screen contact.

When conducting the test it is wise to expose a number of cassettes at the same time, but they must always be of the same speed class. Increasing the numbers saves time and also reduces any chance of errors due to variations in output of the X-ray set. The control cassette will act as confirmation of reproducibility.

Test method

The test tool is placed on top of the cassette and the beam is centred to the centre of the cassette and test tool. The film is exposed using 50 kV, 1.00 or 1.5 mm focal spot, a distance of 1.5 m and sufficient mAs to produce a density of between 2.00 and 3.00. The film is processed in the normal way and viewed at a distance of 4 m.

The important points to note in this test are as follows:

- 50 kV is used, as greater than 55 kV will cause significant over-penetration of the metal

- The density which must be achieved = 2–3 as this is used for the speed measurements as well

- The viewing distance used is 4 m, since it is impossible to see the defects at close range

- Make sure that screens *of the same speed class* are exposed together, along with the control cassette.

When the films are viewed it will be readily apparent which cassettes have a loss of screen contact. A cassette with good screen contact produces films with an overall even density. Poor contact shows up as patches of high density areas (Fig. 10.12).

Cassettes that show poor screen contact in the central area should be rejected. Loss of contact in other areas should be evaluated by the individuals concerned.

Speed tests

A density of greater than 2.0 is produced in the central area of the film; this density measurement also permits a measurement of the relative speed of the screens compared to that of other cassettes exposed using the same exposure factors and conditions.

After the films of the contact test have been reviewed, the density of the central cut-out is measured and all the values recorded. The average is then taken of the highest density values recorded within every speed class. Cassettes which have recorded significantly less than this average density should be rejected on grounds of unacceptable speed loss.

There are two main objections to this test:

1. The first is that exposing at different positions in the X-ray beam can cause variations in exposure.

The only way to overcome this would be to expose a single cassette at a time, on a rotating turntable, so that the cassette was exposed north, south, east and west to the X-ray beam. This is, to say the least, very time-consuming, costly and tedious, but it does represent the most accurate way of testing.

One way to reduce this work would be to take the precaution outlined earlier, whereby a note is kept of the position of every cassette in the X-ray beam. Noticeable errors, e.g. anode heel effect, will show up as consistent errors by virtue of position.

2. The second is the 'decision point' for rejection on grounds of speed.

Perhaps the safest decision to be made is to take an average of two speed classes, e.g. class 100 (universal) and class 200 (special). If the densities recorded on any class 200 approach class 100 densities, then the cassette can safely be

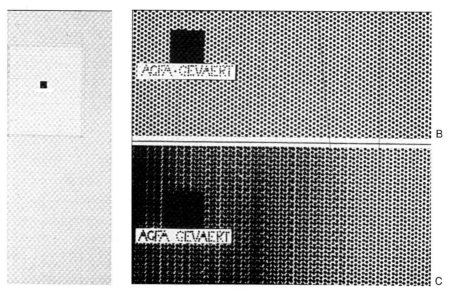

Fig. 10.12 Results from a radiographic test grid: (A) 17″ × 14″ test grid; (B) radiograph produced in a cassette with good screen contact; (C) radiograph produced by a cassette with poor screen contact.

rejected in terms of speed achievement and re-allocated to another room.

Light leakage test

The chances of light leakage occurring in modern cassettes is very slim. Light leakage will be well demonstrated by areas of fogging along the edge of films and therefore it is questionable as to whether it is necessary to perform this British Standard test as a matter of routine as the test is time-consuming to perform.

Test method

Using an 100 W tungsten lamp, expose each edge of the cassette, the front and the back, for 15 min using a distance of 1.22 m. This gives a total of six exposures, taking one and a half hours in total. An edge darkening of less than 3.2 mm on the exposed film is said to be insignificant.

It can now be assumed that all the cassettes have been tested and those which do not conform have been rejected.

THE VIEWING SYSTEM

The remaining part of the chain to check is the viewing boxes themselves. These are still perhaps the most ignored piece of equipment in the department, and yet one of the most important.

VIEWING BOX EVALUATION

The objectives of this test are:

1. To achieve correct and constant light output throughout the department.

2. To achieve the correct balance between viewer light output and the ambient light in the viewing room.

Test equipment

A specifically designed unit which can consist of:

- A hand held-optical recorder
- Laser beam to allow for correct positioning

- A mechanical distance indicator
- Digital display giving a reading in candela per square metre
- The ability to store the data recorded.

The unit is used to assess the overall light intensity from a specific viewing box so that comparisons can be made between viewing boxes to ensure standardisation of viewing facilities.

Cleaning

Viewing boxes must be cleaned both outside and inside as dirt can gather in the inside of a viewing box, causing reduced light output. There are many varieties of antistatic polish available for cleaning viewing box screens.

Colour temperature

Most X-ray films used in the department have a blue base. This base, among other things, produces a much more aesthetically pleasing film. However, a blue base, combined with a yellowish viewing box light, can produce a film which looks very unpleasant and dirty.

It is most important, therefore, to use fluorescent tubes with a wavelength of about 6500 K. This colour temperature is found in tubes with brand names such as 'Northern light' or 'Tropical daylight', both of which produce bright, blue/white light. Colour temperature meters are available, but at a significant cost. The eye can be used as an extremely good judge of the colour temperatures required.

If at any time tubes have to be changed due to discoloration or failure, it is best to change all the tubes in that particular viewing box. In addition, the ideal would be to have all the fluorescent tubes throughout the department exactly the same.

COST-EFFECTIVENESS

Quality assurance should not cost more to perform than it saves. The above series of tests are, to say the least, expensive, as full size film is used for every test. Quality assurance must be cost-effective and this can be achieved in a number of ways.

For example, contact testing should only be undertaken if loss of screen contact is suspected. For routine speed checks, a small size film could be used in the centre of the cassette. This can provide a very accurate method of checking speed, but will not give any guidance in detecting artefacts, etc. However, the UV light will help with this.

When it comes to outright rejection of cassettes it might be worth considering putting all cassettes of the same *measured* speed in the same X-ray room. Many screens can reduce in speed considerably over a period of time. There is no objection at all to matching measured speeds of cassettes together in the same room, as long as the cassettes and screens have passed all other tests. For example, some class 200 screens may actually achieve only class 100 speeds. These, if all other tests are passed, are now used in the room with other *actual* class 100 screens.

The cost of staff to run the quality assurance programme is more difficult to quantify. It is safe to say that a programme will require minutes per day of staff time, rather than hours. Nonetheless, even these figures will add up to a noticeable time in a year. The benefits of such a programme must be weighed carefully.

The decision as to which cassettes to reject is always a problem, due to the cost of any replacement. Low speed screens can be used in the way outlined above; artefacts and contact are much more of a problem. It should of course be noted that rejections due to artefacts and screen contact are the personal decision of the department head.

CONCLUSIONS

It is realised that the ideal and the practical can differ considerably, particularly when the expense of such an exercise is considered. Nevertheless, quality assurance is becoming a very important factor in the modern imaging department.

The advent of the 1985 legal ionising regulations, as opposed to a voluntary code of practice, coupled with the current EC directive, has increased the onus on department heads to prove that equipment is working optimally and correctly.

Quality assurance can be looked upon as another tool in the armoury of an imaging department. It is a means of assuring all interested parties that the equipment within the department is working at optimum efficiency. If records are kept correctly, they will demonstrate the performance of all the equipment used in the department. This certainly enables fault finding to be conducted much more quickly. If a manufacturer has to be contacted because of a fault, a detailed report can be given of the behaviour of the equipment prior to the breakdown.

Quality assurance enables a department to produce high quality radiographs at the minimum dose to the patient and radiographer, at a minimum cost to the department.

REFERENCES

Information from Agfa-Gevaert Limited, Diagnostic Imaging Systems Division, 27 Great West Road, Brentford, Middlesex TW8 9AX

International Standards Organisation 1986 ISO 8374 Photography. Determination of ISO safelight conditions. December 1986 Brussels

Chapter 11
Environmental considerations

INTRODUCTION

Over recent years people have become more environmentally aware, and as a result green issues have taken a place at the top of the nation's agenda, both politically and individually. There will always be new inventions and ideas which further the aim of protecting the environment. Developments such as the advent of cold water processors and low temperature chemicals with the associated reduction in energy usage (and therefore costs), the move towards non-folder wrapped film saving paper, the recycling of chemicals and improved silver recovery have all played their part. Increasing use of computers and imaging plates, which enable the electronic transfer of information can also save on paper and on silver-containing film, not to mention the associated reduction in film processing and therefore chemical usage. However, for many departments, the conventional use of films and film processing still continue to play a major role, and it is with this in mind that this chapter will concentrate on the impact of chemicals in the environment.

ECOLOGICAL CONSIDERATIONS

When the degree of pollution caused by waste water from X-ray film processing is examined it is found that, when compared to other industries, very few problems exist. What follows is a (necessarily) brief description of how to tackle a potentially ecologically unsound process, particularly in less well served urban areas. The following definition, from the *Penguin Dictionary of Science* (1979), is worth bearing in mind as the following pages are read:

The BOD (Biological Oxygen Demand) is a measure of the content of organic matter in water and wastes. It is the amount of oxygen when a sample containing a known mass of oxygen in solution is kept at 20°C for five days. The oxygen is consumed by micro-organisms that feed on the organic matter in the sample.

THE CONTROL OF CHEMICAL POLLUTION

Fortunately, in the past few years there has been a general awareness of how mankind is affecting the environment by the use and abuse of chemicals. Most nations have now taken steps to reduce chemical pollution to acceptable levels. Regrettably, there is still no uniformity of legislation and the regulations controlling pollution vary from country to country. However, the following guidelines will give users a firm basis to start from.

There are three main types of pollution to be considered:

1. Air pollution
2. Soil pollution by solid bodies
3. Water pollution.

AIR AND SOIL POLLUTION

For the first two types, the monitoring of air pollution is discussed under the section on the COSHH Regulations in Chapter 12, and there is sufficient evidence to suggest that for photographic processing soil pollution can be discounted, therefore only the third, water pollution, will be considered in this section.

WATER POLLUTION

A number of factors may be considered when estimating water quality.

Physical pollution factors

These are the factors which can cause water temperatures to rise well above the normal or the water to smell or be badly discoloured. Under normal circumstances the temperature of the liquid waste from X-ray processing does not exceed 37°C. The waste water discharged should not create obnoxious smells nor should discoloration be expected.

Mechanical pollution factors

These are the solids which may be suspended in the effluent. There are no appreciable amounts of solids in the discharge.

pH values

Although the pH of the developer (approximately 10) and the pH of the fixer (approximately 4.5) differ considerably, if they are discharged, with the wash water, through a common discharge pipe, the pH of the effluent will remain within the wanted alkaline range rather than the unwanted acid range.

Oils, fats and inflammable products

These should not be present in effluent and as none are used in the photographic process; they can be discounted in this context.

Dissolved solids

Water authorities analyse for dissolved chemical compounds by using a conductivity test. Examples of dissolved solids identified could include chlorides, sulphates, phosphates, lead, aluminium, etc.

Chemical pollution factors

As far as the photographic process is concerned, this is the most serious area for consideration. Before it is discussed it is important to look at the three separate categories which must be evaluated, namely poisonous materials, biologically oxidisable material and nutrients.

Poisonous materials

These are defined as substances which kill organisms living in the water.

Biologically oxidisable material

When these substances are decomposed by micro-organisms living in the water, oxygen is consumed. This effectively means that aquatic and vegetable life cannot exist.

Nutrients

These are not poisonous, nor do they consume oxygen, but they can upset the ecological balance by promoting the uncontrolled growth of plants and algae.

It is difficult to be precise about what is a toxic substance as almost every substance may be considered toxic if it is present in sufficiently large quantities. Poisons, etc. are easily classified and well documented; the problem occurs when certain chemicals only become toxic when their decomposition products are considered. This can be quantified by considering the biological oxygen demand. This is usually referred to as BOD5 which is expressed as the number of milligrams of oxygen consumed over 5 days per litre of waste water. A sample of water is collected and the oxygen content is measured. The water is then incubated at 20°C for 5 days and the oxygen content is again measured, and by calculating the difference between the two amounts, the BOD can be calculated.

There are certain factors which must be watched in the discharge of photographic waste, but they can be defined and action can be taken to reduce pollution of the environment to a minimum.

If a newly installed processor is connected to a foul sewer the hospital would contact the local water authority for a trade effluent consent. Some rural hospitals have their own treatment works and in this instance the National Rivers Authority should also be involved as the final effluent may enter surface water channels. The trade effluent consent would specify the amount of discharge permitted and this would include the amount of silver in parts per million.

Perspective

It is important to get potential pollution into perspective. The effluent discharged from the processor is diluted many times before leaving the hospital and continues to be diluted in the main sewerage system and by the time it reaches the treatment plant should pose no problems to purification. However, this is no excuse for complacency, and regular monitoring of the efficiency of the processor and the silver recovery system is essential. Special precautions may be necessary if the processor is not connected to a mains sewerage scheme or if discharge is directly into surface water drains. Consultation with the local water authority will always be required during installation.

THE MAIN PHOTOGRAPHIC POLLUTANTS

Metals

Many metallic ions have a serious effect on micro-organisms and fish. Ideally, none of these should be discharged into any sewerage systems.

Silver is the metal most used in the photographic process. When present as a silver ion it is very toxic for most micro-organisms and fish. Silver in the waste water is usually found as a thiosulphate compound from the wash water. This is significantly less toxic than pure silver. In addition, any silver ions present will form almost insoluble salts when combined with chloride, bromide and sulphide ions which are normally present in waste water. The regulations concerning the discharge of silver are discussed in Chapter 12 under the Water Act.

It is imperative that the effluent from any silver recovery unit is monitored on a regular basis to check that no silver is being discharged from the unit. The manager of an imaging department is now responsible for ensuring that if a bulk collection service is used, the company is reputable and, in addition, licensed to dispose of the solutions. These steps can reduce the environmental effect of the discharges of waste solutions but they also give the consumer the added benefit of a return on their investment. If the film used leaves about 5.5 g of silver per litre in the fixing bath, that amounts to about 20 kg of silver available for recovery in the year, assuming 200 working days. Even with the fluctuating values of silver, this still amounts to a potential saving of money.

Possible chemical contaminants

Phenols

Hydroquinone, commonly used as an X-ray developer, is a phenol derivative. One milligram of hydroquinone per litre of water can prove toxic for some fish. If hydroquinone is discharged into a surface water channel it is important that the concentration is kept low.

Ammoniacal nitrogen

In the rapid fixing process, large quantities of ammonium ions are used. However, free ammonia can only occur in an alkaline medium and, although fixer is an acid environment, when mixed with the developer discharge and the waste water the resultant effluent is alkaline.

Organic solvents

These are sometimes used in strongly concentrated processing solutions. Fortunately they have to be diluted to make the processing solution and are then diluted in the waste water until only small traces remain.

Nutrients

Some processing solutions may contain phosphates and nitrates. In processing solutions from the major manufacturers the majority of these radicals have been eliminated.

Oxidising agents

Developer, by its very nature is an oxidising agent. Unfortunately, the presence of developer and sodium sulphite (used to prevent oxidation of the developer) will increase BOD5. Fixer contains thiosulphate, sulphite and possibly, but rarely nowadays, acetate. All of these substances are easily oxidisable.

ACTION

The first steps are taken by the manufacturer of the photographic chemicals. Most manufacturers try to ensure that they use ecologically acceptable chemicals whenever possible. From the consumer's point of view, some forms of process control may be considered necessary. Dilution of the water is not always the answer, but it may well ensure that the waste discharged into surface water channels or into the sewerage system remains within the regulation tolerances. The best option is to try and ensure that the waste water discharge is evenly distributed during the day, even to the extent of installing a collection tank for the waste and then letting the tank drain slowly.

Replenishment of both developer and fixer are the prime causes of contamination of the waste water. Recycling of the developer is difficult as it is not possible selectively to remove the halide ions introduced during development. Even if recycling is undertaken, some replenishment still has to take place, although smaller amounts of chemicals will be used. In either case the best course of action is to ensure that developer replenishment is optimised to the minimum level consistent with good quality results.

Fixer is easier to recycle, but it still requires chemical expertise. As with the developer, the consumer should ensure that the fixer replenishment is kept to a minimum, commensurate with adequate fixation. In Sweden, developer and fixer recyclers are available which allow 40–85% reduction in the volume of developer and fixer being used. Equipment has been successfully installed in British hospitals and there will probably be an increase in demand if the water authorities further reduce the permitted amounts of chemicals which can be discharged in the effluent.

Automatic processors, somewhat surprisingly, help considerably in controlling the equilibrium.

Squeegee rollers reduce carry-over of chemicals, thereby reducing the need for high replenishment rates to restore the pH balance of solutions.

In some circumstances it may be considered necessary to purify and recycle wash water. This can be extremely expensive: for example, when processing was being undertaken on the Alaskan tundra during the construction of the Alaskan oil pipeline, *all* waste was transported out, usually by helicopter, to avoid damaging the delicate natural ecological balance. Again, in Sweden, as a department can only discharge a maximum of 0.5 kg of silver each year, the wash water is recycled. In this instance recycling can achieve a 75% saving in the amount of water used but, in addition, as the water has been heated there is an associated energy saving and the amount of silver discharged in the effluent is negligible.

CONCLUSION

The control of pollution of the environment is in everyone's interest. Most sectors of the community play their part in preserving the environment for future generations. Anyone who is responsible for a process which has the potential for pollution has a duty to reduce that potential to an absolute minimum.

In the case of X-ray processing, the potential hazards are present. Manufacturers play their part by using environmentally friendly chemicals wherever possible and by utilising increasing technological developments. With care, ensuring that the process is working to optimum limits – perhaps using a regular quality assurance programme – pollution can be reduced to an absolute minimum.

REFERENCE

Penguin Dictionary of Science 1979

Chapter 12
Regulations

CHAPTER CONTENTS

INTRODUCTION

As has been stated in the previous chapter, no world-wide uniformity exists concerning the control of pollution or health and safety regulations. It must therefore be emphasised that the following regulations apply to the UK and European Union countries; readers from other countries should check local regulations. The legislation described here has been summarised. Readers are advised to read the chapter in conjunction with the full text of the appropriate regulations, copies of which can be obtained through Stationery Office bookshops.

The regulations listed below are discussed. The legal requirements for dealing with the use and disposal of photographic chemicals are dealt with under this legislation:

- Control of Substances Hazardous to Health (COSHH) Regulations 1999
- Environmental Protection Act (EPA) 1990
- Water Act 1989
- The Chemicals (Hazard Information and Packaging for Supply) Regulations 1994 (amended 99)
- Pollution Prevention and Control Act 1999
- European Packaging Waste Directive 1994

People who regularly work with computer generated images are covered by:

- Health and Safety (Display Screen Equipment) Regulations 1992

The use and disposal of photographic chemicals will be dealt with first.

COSHH REGULATIONS

The COSHH regulations cover many substances which are unlikely to be encountered in modern imaging departments, for example hydrogen cyanide, which is prohibited for use in fumigation in certain circumstances. It must be remembered that the regulations are written for other industries as well as the health sector. It is intended to discuss here only those regulations which do (or may) relate directly to the processing chemicals used in an imaging department.

The COSHH regulations comprise 20 sections but well over half of these are concerned with definitions and the use of the regulations. For example, Regulation 3 makes it clear that the employer is responsible (so far as it is reasonably practicable) for all people who may be affected by substances, whether or not they are employed directly by the employer. In the case of an imaging department, both staff and patients would be covered by the regulations but the employer would not have to apply regulations 10, 11 and 12 to patients as these cover health surveillance, monitoring and training.

Regulations 6–12 relate directly to imaging departments and therefore will be discussed individually.

Regulation 6: Assessment of health risks created by work involving substances hazardous to health

It is required that an assessment of the risks of any substance hazardous to health should be carried out before the employee is asked to work with the substance. Provision is also given to allow the employee to review an assessment if it is thought to be no longer valid.

Regulation 7: Prevention or control of exposure to substances hazardous to health

The emphasis is placed on preventing injury happening and therefore requires that personal protective equipment is provided which is of an approved standard, as outlined in the Personal Protective Equipment (EC Directive) Regulations 1992. This would be used when the manual mixing of chemicals and the wiping up of chemical spillages takes place and would include protective clothing, gloves, eye protectors and respirators. The use of automatic chemical mixers should be considered as these reduce the likelihood of splashing and chemical spillage happening in the first place. Protective clothing should also be used when the processing chemicals are changed and when machines are cleaned.

With regard to inhalation of chemicals, the occupational exposure standards (OESs) must not be exceeded. Lists of OESs are published by the Health and Safety Executive in leaflet EH40 which is updated annually (HSE 2001). Usually two exposure limits are given for each chemical: the long term (8 hours weighted average) and the short term (10 minutes weighted average). The idea behind these figures is that they determine the maximum rate at which a person should be able to tolerate a substance without it affecting their health. As the long term rate is the most strict, this is the rate which is usually quoted although, for example, in the case of glutaraldehyde, only the short term rate is given.

OESs are basically the vapour pressures over a given time and are measured in parts per million. It should be noted that they are therefore concerned with inhalation of substances only. It is possible that a substance could be dangerous as a dust or a vapour but when it is in solution it has a low volatility. It should be remembered that originally processing chemicals were purchased as dry powders and, under these circumstances, hydroquinone, for example, could have posed a hazard. Hydroquinone is now supplied in liquid form (in Part A developer) with a long term exposure limit of 2 mg/m^3 and does not present a significant hazard at the temperatures encountered in radiographic processing. In 2001 the list of OESs was revised and hydroquinone has now been removed from the list.

It is important that the level of exposure to chemicals is kept as low as possible and that the maximum exposure limits are not exceeded. Regulation 7.5.b requires the employer to take action and, as soon as is reasonable, remedy the situation if it is identified that the OES has been exceeded.

One way of helping to reduce the quantity of fumes is by ensuring there is adequate ventilation (in the order of 12–15 air changes per hour) and, if possible, by ducting processors to the outside air. As higher temperatures result in increased evaporation, the use of low temperature and 'low fume' chemicals should be considered for use where appropriate. In addition, good drainage, the proper siting of silver recovery equipment and the safe and correct handling of chemicals all contribute to minimising the amount of chemicals present in the environment.

Regulation 8: Use of control measures

Employers should try to ensure that substances are used in the correct manner but, in addition, employees should ensure that they use the equipment correctly and report any defects to their employer as soon as possible.

Regulation 9: Maintenance, examination and test of control measures

Non-disposable personal protective equipment should be checked by the employer at 'suitable intervals' by thorough examination and, where necessary, tests. A record should be made detailing the date, the examination/test, the results and, if appropriate, any repairs undertaken. These records should be kept for 5 years from the date they were made.

Regulation 10: Monitoring exposure at the workplace

The type of monitoring required under this regulation would be concerned with ensuring that the occupational exposure limits were not breached for those substances present in processing chemicals.

Manufacturers supply health and safety data sheets which provide written information on, for example, the chemicals, their concentration, hazard indication, safe use, storage and first aid/accident action. These data sheets can be used in conjunction with EH40 to determine the long term exposure limits for monitoring purposes. In some instances it is possible to smell a substance at a level much lower than when it is considered to be a hazard while other substances may not have a detectable odour – therefore smell is no substitute for accurate measurement. It is possible to use portable gas detection equipment, particularly for the detection of sulphur dioxide which can give an indication of the general level of fumes in a department. As this type of equipment tends to err on the high side, any reading below the OES can be regarded as being safe.

Some companies provide a service for more accurate measurements by sampling the atmosphere using special absorbents and then analysing the sample by using, for example, gas chromatography. Records of monitoring should be kept for at least 5 years unless they relate to identifiable employees in which case they should be kept for 30 years.

Regulation 11: Health surveillance

Health surveillance should take place if an adverse health effect may be related to the exposure. This may become a requirement with regard to such chemicals as glutaraldehyde (short term OES 0.2 parts per million) but as some manufacturers are now producing glutaraldehyde-free developer this may not be necessary. Monoethylene glycol (long term OES 23 parts per million) (antifreeze) used to be used extensively as a solvent for phenidone but it is now considered to be dangerous in vapour form and therefore has been replaced either by diethylene glycol (23 parts per million) – which gained notoriety as an illegal addition to wine – or monopropylene glycol (150 parts per million), the latter being the least dangerous chemical.

Therefore, depending on the processing chemicals used, health surveillance may or may not be necessary. If monitoring is needed it should take place at least every 12 months and records should be kept for 30 years.

Regulation 12: Information, instruction and training

It is the responsibility of the employer to provide instruction and training in the safe use of processing chemicals including information about the health hazards and the precautions which should be taken. In addition, if an OES is exceeded, the employee (or their representative) should be informed.

In summary, it should be remembered that imaging chemicals are no more dangerous than many other substances that can be found in the home or in industry. Risks occur due to inhalation, exposure to the eyes, absorption through the skin, injection and ingestion. The COSHH regulations are designed to promote safe working practices including monitoring and training in the use of substances which may be hazardous to health. The accurate implementation of the regulations should be of benefit to all.

ENVIRONMENTAL PROTECTION ACT 1990

This act first introduced the concept of 'integrated pollution control' which covers the discharge of certain substances to land, water or air. This area does not appear to have significant implications for imaging departments. However, also included in the Act is a 'duty of care', the most pertinent aspect of which is that the person disposing of waste should only transfer it to those who are authorised to receive it. Therefore care must be taken to check that those who receive departmental waste, for example silver recovery firms, are licensed to dispose of the product.

WATER ACT 1989

As hospitals have now lost their Crown immunity it will become necessary for them to obtain a trade effluent discharge consent. The amount charged for this consent is decided by the strength and volume of the effluent and tends to vary between water authorities, as does the permitted level of silver in the effluent. Many Western economies (and some water authorities) set the silver level at 2 parts per million but as there are large variations throughout the country it is safer to check with the local water authority as to the levels they permit.

The 23 most dangerous chemical pollutants are on what is referred to as the 'red list' and these are the chemicals that are currently receiving the most attention. Silver appears on the next list (grey) and it is predicted that controls on effluent may become much tighter. This tightening of the regulations may well mean that developer, fixer and even wash water (which contains silver) may have to be collected for disposal rather than put down the drain.

It is possible to recycle developer, fixer and wash water. This can result in a dramatic reduction of the silver content of the effluent and additionally has the advantage of saving the amount of chemicals and water used; the associated heating costs can also be reduced along with a reduction in the cost of the processor chemical bill.

Equipment is available which uses the product of fixer recycling and mixes it with used developer in such a way as to produce a fairly neutral pH and avoid the production of sulphur dioxide and ammonia. The resultant chemical is then diluted with water and discharged to waste. It has to be said that there are critics of this system who say that the chemicals are still being discharged and therefore this is just a way of getting round trade consents.

CHEMICALS (HAZARD INFORMATION AND PACKAGING FOR SUPPLY) REGULATIONS 1994 (AMENDED 99) (CHIP)

These regulations cover such topics as:

- The classification of dangerous substances
- The symbols used for dangerous substances
- The preparation of dangerous substances

- Information for safety data sheets
- The labelling of substances
- The British and international standards for child resistant fastenings and tactile warning devices.

The regulations are for manufacturers and suppliers. It is a means of classifying substances that may be a hazard during normal handling and use. In the guidance notes care has been taken to show the difference between hazard and risk, hazard being defined as 'the inherent properties of a chemical' and risk 'the probability of the hazardous properties of the chemical causing harm to people or the environment'.

Substances on the list include:

- Acetic acid
- EDTA
- Glutaraldehyde
- Hydroquinone
- 1-phenyl-3-pyrazolidone (Phenidone)
- Potassium carbonate
- Potassium hydroxide
- Potassium sulphite
- Sodium hydroxide.

The label is intended to provide information about the hazards and the precautions which can be taken when using the substance. These include:

- Storage
- Clothing to be worn during preparation
- Correct handling
- Disposal of material.

It is therefore important that all labels are carefully read and that the instructions and advice contained in them are followed.

POLLUTION PREVENTION AND CONTROL ACT 1999: IMPLEMENTING EUROPEAN COUNCIL POLLUTION PREVENTION DIRECTIVE 96/61/EC

This directive follows the principle that the polluter pays and encourages the prevention of pollution. It is concerned with pollution into the air, water and the soil and covers both old and new buildings. Its aim is to integrate all existing legislation. Annex IV mentions:

- The use of low waste technology
- The use of less hazardous substances
- Recovery and recycling
- The nature effect and volume of emissions
- The reduction of the impact of emissions on the environment.

The reader is recommended to look at the full document which is available on the internet (http://www.europa.eu.int/eur-lex/en/lif/dat/1996/en396L0061.html).

EUROPEAN PACKAGING AND PACKAGING WASTE DIRECTIVE 1994 94/62/EC

This directive sets targets for the reuse and recycling of plastics, paper, cardboard, metal and glass. At the time of writing, the target for packaging is that 50–65% of waste should be recovered and up to 70% of commercial waste. However, an amendment to the directive is expected in 2001 and it is thought that the targets will be changed.

HEALTH AND SAFETY (DISPLAY SCREEN EQUIPMENT) REGULATIONS 1992

The regulations have been introduced because if display screen equipment is used for long periods of time the operator may experience musculoskeletal problems, eye fatigue and stress. The regulations therefore have a preventative role by introducing the need to provide correctly designed office equipment. Information is provided in the guidelines concerning the display screen, keyboard, work desk or surface and type of work chair. In addition, the work environment is discussed with relation to the space provided, lighting, reflection and glare, noise, heat and humidity. Lastly, the type of work being undertaken and the software used are also covered.

These regulations cover employees who use display screen equipment for a significant part of their normal work. They can be defined as individuals who use the equipment daily and for continuous spells of an hour or more at a time. It is important that the regulations are studied carefully if an employer feels that some of their staff may come into this category. With the increasing use of visual display units in imaging departments many more staff will be covered by these regulations.

The key duties of employers are as follows:

- To identify areas where display screen equipment is used

- To identify which staff use the equipment and for how long

- To assess the risks to users (if any) and reduce the risks where appropriate

- To ensure that any new workstations meet the health and safety requirement (workstations existing at the time the regulations appeared should have been brought up to standard by 31 December 1996)

- To make sure that staff have adequate breaks and changes of activity

- To provide users with eye and eyesight tests, if appropriate

- To ensure that any users receive adequate training and information concerning safe working practices.

CONCLUSION

Legislation is introduced to ensure good and safe working practices and is therefore of long term benefit for all concerned. Every employee should be aware of what constitutes safe working practices and should be aware that bad practice can harm not only themselves but, where the discharge of waste is concerned, potentially their colleagues, friends and relatives in the community as well.

REFERENCES

Chemicals (Hazard Information and Packaging for Supply) Regulations 1994 (amended 99) Statutory Instrument 1994 No. 3247, The Stationery Office, ISBN 0110438779 (full text on website)
European Council Pollution Prevention Directive 96/61/EC. Can be consulted at http://www.europa.eu.int/eur-lex/en/lif/dat/1996/en396L0061.html
European Packaging Waste Directive 1994 European Parliament and Council Directive 94/62/EC 20 Dec 1994 on packaging and packaging waste
Health and Safety Executive 1993 EH40
Health and Safety Executive 1993 Health and Safety (Display screen equipment) Regulations 1992, HSE information sheet No. 5

Health and Safety Executive 2001 Occupational exposure standards. EH40/2001
HMSO 1989 Water Act
HMSO 1990 Environmental Protection Act
Stationery Office Ltd, Personal Protective Equipment (EC Directive) Regulations 1992, ISBN 0110 252527
Stationery Office Ltd, Pollution Prevention and Control Act 1999, ISBN 0 10 542499
Stationery Office 1999 Control of Substances Hazardous to Health Regulations 1999, The Health and Safety Executive, Statutory Instrument 437 1999, ISBN 011 082 087 8

Further information

FURTHER READING

Further information is available from the following publications and websites:

Agfa Gevaert NV 1978 For a better environment. General information. Agfa Gevaert Ltd, 27 Great West Road, Brentford, Middlesex TW8 9AX

Agfa Gevaert NV 1978 For a better environment. Hints for the X-ray sector. Agfa Gevaert Ltd, 27 Great West Road, Brentford, Middlesex TW8 9AX

Care Geof/Photosol 1992 Ultimate waste disposal. Photosols Ltd, 15 Bakers Court, Paycocke Road, Basildon, Essex SS14 3EH

Care Geof/Photosol 1992 X-ray chemistry and the environment. Photosols Ltd, 15 Bakers Court, Paycocke Road, Basildon, Essex SS14 3EH

Graham D 1996 Principles of radiological physics. Churchill Livingstone, Edinburgh

Health and Safety Executive 1992 Display screen equipment work: guidance on regulations

Health and Safety Executive 1992 Working with VDUs

Health and Safety Executive 1993 EH40

Health and Safety Executive 1993 Health and Safety (Display screen equipment) Regulations 1992. HSE information sheet No. 5

Health and Safety Executive 2001 EH40/2001

HMSO 1988 Control of Substances Hazardous to Health Regulations 1988

HMSO 1989 Water Act

HMSO 1990 Environmental Protection Act

Hogg P 1993 Remote computing – the shape of things to come? Radiography Today, July 1993

HSC Approved guide to the classification and labelling of substances and preparations dangerous for supply, 3rd edn. Health and Safety Executive 6/97

http://europa.eu.int/eur-lex/en/lif/dat/1994/en_394L0062.html

http://medical.nema.org/dicom.html

http://www.europa.eu.int/eur-lex/en/lif/dat/1996/en396L0061.html

http://www.hse.gov.uk

http://www.rsna.org/IHA/qa.shtml

Photosol 1992 Fumes from X-ray chemistry. Photosols Ltd, 15 Bakers Court, Paycocke Road, Basildon, Essex SS14 3EH

Photosol 1997 Ultimate waste disposal. Photosols Ltd, 15 Bakers Court, Paycocke Road, Basildon, Essex SS14 3EH

Photosol 1997 X-ray chemistry and the environment. Photosols Ltd, 15 Bakers Court, Paycocke Road, Basildon, Essex SS14 3EH

Wheeler Graham 2000 A new concept in PACS, Everything On-Line Laser Lines Ltd

www.agfa.co.uk

www.kodak.com/go/health

www.medical.agfa.com

www.metafix.co.uk

www.r2tech.com

www.radin.de

PRODUCT INFORMATION/MANUFACTURERS

Agfa Gevaert Ltd, 27 Great West Road, Brentford, Middlesex TW8 9AX

Data General Ltd, Data General Tower, Great West Road, Brentford, Middlesex TW8 9AN

Fuji 1993 Data Management System. Product information.

Fuji Photo Film (UK) Ltd, 125 Finchley Road, London NW3 6HY

Knight Systems, Scientific House, Rectory Farm Road, Sompting, Lancing, West Sussex BN15 0DP

Kodak Ltd, PO Box 66, Station Road, Hemel Hempstead, Herts HP1 1JU

Konica (UK) Ltd, Plane Tree Crescent, Feltham, Middlesex TW13 7HD

Lanmark 2000 Product information leaflet. Lanmark, PO Box 317, Beaconsfield, Bucks HP9 2LR

Laser Lines Ltd, Beaumont Close, Banbury, Oxon OX16 7TQ

Medical Imaging Systems, 12 Kingsbury Trading Estate, Church Lane, Kingsbury NW9 8AU

Metafix UK Ltd, 1–3 Enterprise Road, Raunds, Northants NN9 6JE

Photosols Ltd, 15 Bakers Court, Paycocke Road, Basildon, Essex SS14 3EH

Siemens 1993 Sienet product information brochure. Siemens Medical Engineering, Siemens House, Oldbury, Bracknell, Berks RG12 8FZ

Southern Scientific Ltd, Scientific House, Rectory Farm Road, Sompting, Lancing, West Sussex BN15 0DP

X-Rite, The Acumen Centre, First Avenue, Pointon, Cheshire SK12 1FJ

Appendices

Glossary of computer buzzwords

The following glossary is by no means comprehensive, but it contains many of the buzzwords in current use.

Access time   The time taken for the computer to get information from a storage device, e.g. disk or tape.

Address   A number which designates a particular storage area in the memory of the computer.

Algorithm   Logical steps which define how a problem can be solved.

Analogue   Represents a quantity changing in steps which are continuous, as opposed to *digital* which is in discrete steps.

A voltmeter with a needle pointer is an *analogue* device. It can record an infinitely variable number of readings. A voltmeter with a digital display is limited to the number of steps it is allowed to display, i.e. it is a *digital* device.

Analogue to digital converter   A device which converts analogue signals into digital signals which can be understood by the computer.

ASCII   The **A**merican **S**tandard **C**ode for **I**nformation **I**nterchange. This code defines the decimal and binary code of all the characters stored in the computer.

For example:

[Decimal]	[Binary]	[Character]
115	01110011	s
34	00100010	"
68	01000100	D

Attachment   A document sent with an e-mail.

BASIC   A high level language for computers and almost universally used for home computers. It is an acronym of **B**eginners **A**ll-purpose **S**ymbolic **I**nstruction **C**ode.

Baud   This is the unit for measuring the rate at which data are transmitted or received.

Binary   A system of counting to base two, i.e. generating figures with only 1 or 0.

Bit   The smallest unit of data in a computer. It is a contraction of **BI**nary digi**T**.

Booting   Starting up the computer by loading it with its starting instructions.

Bps   **B**its **p**er **s**econd, the rate information is transferred between computers.

Bounce   The automatic return of e-mail.

Bubblejet printer   This printer is ribbonless, the ink reaches the paper in electrostatically formed bubbles and prints very quietly. Slightly higher resolution (± 15%) than an inkjet printer may be expected from this technology, pioneered by Canon. Print speed is similar to an inkjet and, like an inkjet printer, the new ink cartridge contains a new printhead.

Buffer   An area which stores information at one rate and releases it at a slower rate to another device.

For example, a buffer can be sited between a computer (fast) and a printer (which is significantly slower). Data can then be passed at a fast rate and stored in the buffer until the printer can print the data. The computer is thus freed for further work much more rapidly.

Bug   A problem in the computer or (usually) in the program.

Bus   A semi-standard connector to the computer through which all data are passed to an external device.

Byte   The number of bits which are needed to form a single character. This is usually 8.

1 kilobyte (1 K) is not 1000 bits but 1024 bits. This is because of binary arithmetic: 1 kilobyte is $2 \times 2 \times 2 \times 2 \times 2 \times 2 \times 2 \times 2 \times 2 \times 2$, or 2 to the power 10.

Centronics   A type of standard interface between computer and peripheral.

The standard defines the plug and socket sizes and how the data are transmitted between the computer and peripheral.

CD ROM   A **c**ompact **d**isc with **r**ead **o**nly **m**emory.

CP/M   One of the most common 'universal' languages.

A number of computers speak BASIC but, as in all languages, there are many dialects. This means that there are very few computers on which it is possible to use a program from another computer of a different make.

CP/M is a disk-based language which tries to rectify this. Most computers running CP/M can interchange programs quite easily.

CPS   **C**haracters **P**er **S**econd, a measure of the speed of data output.

CPU   **C**entral **P**rocessing **U**nit: the core of the computer.

Chip   A piece of silicon which contains the microcircuitry which operates the computer. Gallium arsenide is also used.

Cursor   A flashing marker on the screen which indicates where the next character is to be inserted.

Daisy wheel printer   A high-quality printer, in which the printing head consists of characters arranged on a series of 'petals' arranged in a circle.

Data compression   The reduction in size of information to decrease transferred film size.

Data Protection Act   Only registered users can hold information about individuals on computer and all patients have a right under this act to see any records concerning themselves or their treatment.

Database   Software designed to store information in a systematic way, and at the same time to allow easy retrieval and manipulation of all data.

Debugging   The correction and, much more importantly, the finding of errors or bugs in a program.

DICOM   **D**igital **I**maging and **CO**mmunications in **M**edicine, a project to bring manufacturers together to agree standardisation in computerised image transfer and communications.

Digital   See *analogue*.

Disk   A circular plastic disc coated with magnetic material used for storing data. Disks are usually high speed devices.

Domain name   The location of an organisation or individual on the internet.

Dongle   Any device used to protect software from piracy.

Download   To transfer information from one computer to another.

DOS   **D**isk **O**perating **S**ystem. This is the software which controls the disk drive.

Dot matrix   A square or rectangle of dots which, given instructions by the computer, forms a character. Usually refers to a printing head, but could refer (for example) to the construction of a character on the screen.

Dot matrix printer   A printer which produces characters or images by a matrix head striking a ribbon (similar to a typewriter) and producing characters made up of a series of dots. They range from 9 pin heads through 24 pin up to as many as 48 pin and can be the most inexpensive of all the printers. As these are impact printers they can have high noise levels. The image is usually fairly coarse, particularly when enlarged, as typical resolution expected from this type of printer would be approximately 180 dpi (dots per inch).

DVD   **D**igital **V**ersatile **D**isc, a disc capable of storing more information at a higher quality than a compact disc (CD).

Editing   Altering the text or program.

eMail   This is an electronic mail system. Its current uses include sending imaging reports and pathology reports directly to GP surgeries from one computer to another via Healthlink. It may also be used by GPs for the direct referral of patients for examinations.

Emulation   There is a proliferation of computer printers. Some standards have been adopted by the large manufacturers. Epson (printer manufacturers) wrote an ESC (Epson Standard Code) sequence which is a control for dot matrix printers. Many other manufacturers *emulate* this ESC sequence to make sure that their printers work successfully. Laser printers usually emulate the Hewlett Packard standard. Unfortunately computer types proliferate, unable to read one another's disks, etc. For example, different high level languages are used by: IBM (and clones), Acorn, Atari, Amiga, CP/M (which was initially conceived as the universal language of computers). Some manufacturers emulate another operating system so that they can read the information stored on (otherwise incompatible) disks.

Encryption   A method of coding data to prevent unauthorised access to the information.

EPROM   **E**rasable **P**rogrammable **R**ead **O**nly **M**emory. A memory store which can be programmed but erased, if washed, by UV light.

Erasable optical disks (Magneto-optical disks or MO disks)   These read *and* write optical disks are becoming more and more available. They combine magnetic and optical techniques. One typical technique, when the disk is re-used, is to heat the magnetic layer (with the ubiquitous laser) to the point where its coercivity drops, thus making erasure of magnetic information very easy with low magnetic fields. This layer – made of terbium, iron and cobalt – cools very quickly, regaining high coercivity when the heat source is withdrawn. On the next rotation of the disk, new information is magnetically recorded. On the third rotation the laser reads the information, i.e. light which has been polarised when shone through the magnetic layer (due to the Kerr effect), and checks if this information is correct.

A recent type of erasable optical disk is the 'phase change drive'. This disk uses a heat-deformable crystalline surface material which can exist in two states – reflective and nonreflective. Like the 'pits' on a music CD, these areas provide the 0 and 1s needed for data transmission when 'playedback' by the laser. This type of read/write disk is capable of being used up to 1 000 000 times.

FAQ   **F**requently **A**sked **Q**uestion.

File   Information stored on disk or cassette.

Firewall   A security system to prevent unauthorised access to information.

Firmware   Software, but stored on a chip.

Floppy disk   A flexible disk (see disk) usually 3.5 inches in diameter.

Flowchart   A diagrammatic representation of a computer program.

FORTRAN   A programming language which is between BASIC and machine code in difficulty.

Gate   A gate performs a single logical operation when subjected to a number of inputs. It is the basis of all computer operations.

Golf ball   A printing head usually found on electronic typewriters. Shaped like a golf ball, with printing characters arranged around its surface, the ball rotates very rapidly to present different characters to the typewriter ribbon.

Graphical User Interface (GUI)   It was generally recognised that when a PC was controlled by typing the commands in via DOS it was hardly satisfactory, requiring deep knowledge of the DOS. It was decided to produce a graphical user interface which enabled the operator to use the computer intuitively via graphics (pictures) showing programs to run, directories they are kept in, etc. The best-known GUI is 'Windows' from Microsoft.

Graphics   This can refer to a number of things:
1. Computerised 'drawing', known as CAD (Computer Aided Drawing).
2. The ability of the computer to produce preprogrammed graphic characters.
3. The mode the computer has to be placed in prior to drawing graphics.

Graphics tablet   A piece of equipment that can digitise drawing or graphs ready for input into the computer.

Handshake   An electronic signal which indicates the end of the passage of data from the computer.

Hard copy   The paper printout of the program or screen display.

Hardware   The mechanical and electronic part of the equipment.

Healthlink   A centralised, data communications network. It enables authorised users to exchange documents and information cheaply and efficiently.

Heuristic   A 'trial and error' method of trying to solve a problem.

Hexadecimal   A mathematical system which employs 16 digits from 0 to 9 plus A, B, C, D, E, F. For example, hexadecimal 24A is equal to decimal 570.

Icon   A relatively new move in computers to make them more 'user friendly'.

An icon is displayed on the screen, e.g. a waste basket. This indicates that, if this icon is selected, the software is programmed to dump the data, as if it were a real waste basket.

Initialise   At the beginning of computation all variables are given specific values in the program.

For example: A = 1, B = 7, C = 4.

In this example, A, B and C are the variables initialised at those values.

Inkjet printer   This printer does not use a ribbon; the ink is sprayed on through very fine jets, building up the characters or images in very fine dots virtually silently. Typically, resolutions of 300×300 dpi can be expected from this technology, pioneered by Hewlett Packard. Printed page production is relatively slow, of the order of 30–60 seconds. When a new ink cartridge is inserted it contains a new printhead.

Intelligent peripheral   A keypad linked to a computer that can act as a computer in its own right.

Interface   The connection from the computer to other hardware, allowing free communication between the two.

ISDN   Integrated Services Digital Network, a set of standards for the transfer of digital information over a telephone wire and other media.

ISP   Internet Service Provider, a company that allows connection to the internet.

Iteration   To repeatedly execute an instruction in a program. For example:

100 FOR X = 1 TO 200: NEXT X

In line 100, the routine has been iterated 200 times.

Internet   World-wide network of computers.

Intranet   Network of computers within a specific area, e.g. a hospital or group of hospitals.

Java   A programming language that works on all computer systems.

Jukebox   An electromechanical device for handling large numbers of optical computer disks to enable the rapid retrieval of archived data.

Laser printer   Sometimes referred to as a 'page printer'. It is ribbonless and does not use ink cartridges but 'toner'. The characters or images are built up by being scanned by a laser and then toner is fused onto the paper. Fast (about 4–10 pages a minute) and quiet with what can be very high resolution (up to 600×600 dpi).

Light pen   A device, shaped like a pen, which interfaces with a computer screen and enables the computer to know which part of the screen is being pointed to.

LISP   LISt Processor language. A language used a great deal in artificial intelligence research. It is a high level language.

LOGO   A high level language usually used in schools to introduce primary school children to computers.

LSI   Large Scale Integration. A means of packing large numbers of electronic circuits into small chips.

Soon to be followed by VLSI, or Very Large Scale Integration.

Machine code   The language the computer can understand directly.

In a high level language, commands are simplified into pure English. In machine code, all instructions are written in binary.

Mainframe   A large computer, usually the centre of a system. Intelligent peripherals can then be attached to this.

Menu   A set of choices presented in a program.

For example:
1. New patient
2. Alter patient details
3. Next appointment
4. Report details
ENTER NUMBER OF CHOICE.

Microprocessor   A very complex integrated circuit that can be pre-programmed to perform a variety of tasks.

MIME   Multipurpose Internet Mail Extensions, a method of sending binary objects by e-mail.

Modem   MOdulator-DEModulator. A device, also known as an acoustic coupler, which allows the computer to transmit data down a conventional telephone line.

Monitor   A device very similar to a television, but which receives video signals directly from the computer, rather than RE-modulated signals, giving much more accurate resolution.

Mouse   Again, a device for making the computer more 'user friendly'. Instead of accessing the computer via a keypad, the mouse is used by rolling the device across a desk top. This, in turn, moves a cursor to icon displays on the screen.

MSX   A new standard for home computers based on Microsoft Extended Basic.

This standard specifies minimum capacity, graphic display size and fittings for peripherals. Hopefully the MSX standard means that any program written for one MSX computer will be interchangeable with another make of MSX computer.

Network   A system, usually connected by telephone line, which interconnects a number of computers enabling multiway communication within the network.

OCR   Optical Character Recognition. A means of the computer directly reading printed or written characters.

OCR was meant originally to be used with post codes, but it constantly runs into a classic computer problem known as the 'B8 problem'. In other words, the computer has great difficulty in recognising the difference between B and 8, apart from problems of handwriting differences.

Output   Data and information leaving a computer. This data can then be sent to a display screen, printer or another computer.

PACS   Picture Archiving and Communications System, for allowing transfer of images and data across the intranet. For example radiographs and reports.

PASCAL   A high level language for computers.

Passwords   Entry is forbidden into many computer controlled systems unless a particular password has been entered. This provides fairly good security and virtually stops unwarranted interference with the data. Passwords are frequently graded, so that limited access to the system is allowed by some passwords but unlimited access is provided by other passwords.

PC: Personal computer   This acronym denotes the ubiquitous standard for personal computers. Initially developed by IBM as an AT (Advanced Technology) and the XT (eXtended Technology) computers. The creation of these computers spawned a major new industry, the 'cloning' of PCs.

Peripheral Any device attached to a computer, e.g. a printer or modem.

Pixel Picture cell. A pixel is the smallest number of dots which can be used by a character on the display screen.

It can also be used to define the resolution of a system by describing the resolution of a matrix in pixels, i.e. 1200 × 1200 gives a resolution of 1200 separate points horizontally and vertically.

POP Post Office Protocol, an e-mail system.

Program A set of written instructions for the computer.

PROM Programmable Read Only Memory. A specially prepared chip which can be programmed, turning it into a Read Only Memory.

Protocol Written standards for the transfer of information between different computers.

RAM Random Access Memory. This is the part of the memory of the computer which can be accessed by the user.

The amount of RAM available determines how much data can be stored by the user. It is usually shown as 16K, 32K, 48K or 64K in the smaller home computers.

In the bigger business type computers, many hundreds if not thousands of kilobytes may be quoted.

Real time Usually defined as a computer controlling, or recording, events as they are actually happening.

Remark Usually seen in a program as REM. This instruction is ignored by the computer, but enables the user to add comments in plain English.

RGB input This refers to a colour input on a *monitor*. The signal from the computer or video apparatus is taken by the monitor as a basic Red, Green and Blue input.

ROM Read Only Memory: the pre-programmed part of the computer which enables it to run programs. While it may be accessible to the user, it cannot be altered.

RS 232 A type of standard interface between computer and peripheral. The standard defines the plug and socket sizes and how the data is transmitted between the computer and peripheral.

Scanners Computers can use a device which enables documents, pictures, etc. to be scanned and the resultant scan held as a digital image.

Scrolling The movement of text or data on the display screen. Scrolling can be upwards, downwards or even sideways.

Search engine A database of key words that internet users can access to find information on the web.

Server A method of enabling computers to communicate with each other either by using another computer or software on a computer.

Service providers Organisations that offer connections to the internet.

Software The programs run by the computer.

Spam Unrequested e-mail – usually advertising products or services.

Speech recognition A software development allowing computers to be operated by human voice commands.

Speech synthesis A software development allowing the computer to 'talk' to the user.

Spreadsheet A program which allows forecasting and financial planning. It can be thought of as a massive financial ledger in which, if any variable is altered, the effects throughout the ledger can be demonstrated and the figures changed throughout the ledger without further input from the user.

Sprite A user-generated character, much used in game playing. The sprite can be kept moving at a certain speed by the computer, independent of any other movement on the screen.

SSL Secure Socket Layer, a method of verifying the identity of system users and web sites.

Statement An instruction in a program.

Subroutine A self-contained part of a program which can be returned to time and time again within a program.

Syntax error Two words which are shown on the display when an incorrect input or statement has been made.

Teletex The sending of documents at high speed electronically.

Teletext The non-interactive public information service on television. The BBC transmits Ceefax.

Time bomb A device used by some software suppliers to prevent piracy of programs, which is a growing menace in the computer world. The software is protected by a certain phrase or code which can be removed by the legitimate supplier. If it is not, after a period of use the software is so arranged that it will wipe itself out and erase all the company records.

Turnkey A term used to denote a company which will provide all the necessary software and hardware plus back-up support to enable the user to 'turn a key' and use the equipment.

Turtle A wheeled mechanical device, used for graphics, attached to a computer via cables. Initially associated with *LOGO* where the Turtle would draw its path (the Turtle Trail) across paper.

URL Uniform Resource Locator, the address of internet files.

USB Universal Serial Bus, the sockets connecting hardware to a computer.

VDU Video Display Unit.

Virus A program introduced into the computer system to corrupt the main program. New disks (including computer games) should always be checked before being used in the hospital computer system.

VOXEL A *pixel* but in three dimensions.

WAP Wireless Application Protocol, a standard to allow text messages from the web to be available to mobile phones.

Winchester disk A very large capacity *hard* disk, as opposed to *floppy*. The disk is housed in a hermetically sealed container, as any ingress of dust or dirt, no matter how microscopic, could possibly destroy very large amounts of data.

Word processor A combination of computer, software and printer enabling the user to produce high quality text which can be manipulated electronically before being committed to paper.

WORM An acronym for Write Once Read Many. It is used in the context of optical disks which are used once to receive data for archiving and can subsequently be read as often as is required.

WWW World Wide Web, an information and resource centre for the internet.

Zap A small alteration to a program.

2

Abbreviations

AFW	Alternative folder wrapped (film)
Ag^+	Silver ion
AgBr	Silver bromide
AgCl	Silver chloride
AgI	Silver iodide
$AgNO_3$	Silver nitrate
Ag_2S	Silver sulphide
$AlCl_3$	Aluminium chloride
$Al_2(SO_4)_3$	Aluminium sulphate
ANSI	American National Standards Institute
ASCII	American Standard Code for Information Interchange
BaFCl	Barium fluorochloride
BaFCl.Eu	Barium fluorochloride with europium activator
BOD	Biochemical oxygen demand
Br^-	Bromide ion
BS	British Standard
c	Velocity
CAD	Computer aided drawing
$CaWO_4$	Calcium tungstate
$C_6H_4O_2$	Quinone
$C_6H_6O_2$	Hydroquinone
COSHH	Control of Substances Hazardous to Health
CRT	Cathode ray tube
CT	Computed tomography
Cv	Critical value
D	Density
Dev	Developer
DIN	Deutsche Industrie Normen
Dmax	Maximum density
e^-	Electron
E	Energy or exposure
EDTA	Ethylene diamine tetra-acetic acid
EPA	Environmental Protection Act
Eu	Europium
EV	Exposure value
F	Field size
f	Frequency of radiation
ffd	Focus-film distance
FN	False negative
fod	Focus-object distance
FP	False positive
FW	Folder wrapped (film)
$\bar{G}$	Average gradient
Gbytes	Gigabytes
Gd	Gadolinium
Gd_2O_2S	Gadolinium oxysulphide
$Gd_2O_2S.Tb$	Gadolinium oxysulphide with terbium activator
H^+	Hydrogen ion
h	Planck's constant
HBr	Hydrogen bromide
H & D	Hurter and Driffield (curve in sensitometry)
HIS	Hospital information system
HSE	Health and Safety Executive
Hz	Hertz
I	Intensity
Io	Incident light
IEP	Isoelectric point
IF	Intensifying factor
in	Inch
ISO	International Organisation for Standardisation
J	Joules
K	Degrees Kelvin (= degrees centigrade + 273)
KBr	Potassium bromide
KeV	Kiloelectron volt
KNO_3	Potassium nitrate
K_2SO_3	Potassium sulphite
kV	Kilovolt
Kw	Equilibrium constant of water
λ	Wavelength
l	Litre
La	Lanthanum
LaOBr	Lanthanum oxybromide
LaOBr.Tb	Lanthanum oxybromide with terbium activator
LASER	Light amplification by stimulation emission of radiation
LBD	Light beam diaphragm
LCD	Liquid crystal display
LED	Light emitting diodes
logIt	Logarithm of light intensity (intensity × time)
lp mm^{-1}	Line pairs per millimetre
lux	1 Lumen per square metre
μ	Micron
m	Metre
M	Mega
mAs	Milliamps × seconds
Mbytes	Megabytes
MHz	Megahertz
mol	Mole (molecular weight in grams)
MRI	Magnetic resonance imaging

MTF	Modulation transfer function	RF	Radio frequency
Na	Absorption efficiency	RGB	Red, green, blue (output)
$Na_2S_2O_3$	Sodium thiosulphate	RIS	Radiology information system
Na_2SO_3	Sodium sulphite	ROC	Receiver operating characteristics
ND	Net density		
Ne	Emission efficiency	s	Seconds
$(NH_2CH_2COOH)_n$	Gelatine	SDT	Signal detection theory
$(NH_4)_2S_2O_3$	Ammonium thiosulphate		
Ni	Conversion efficiency	θ	Variable field compensation factor
NIF	Non-interleaved film	t	Time
nm	Nanometres	T	Transmitted (light)
Nt	Total efficiency	Tb	Terbium
		TDS	Total dissolved solids
OES	Occupational exposure standard	TiO_2	Titanium dioxide
OH^-	Hydroxyl ion	TN	True negative
Ortho	Orthochromatic	TP	True positive
		TRIR	Total radiation intensity range
P	Phenidone or phosphor		
PACS	Picture archiving and communication system	Ug	Geometric unsharpness
		Um	Movement unsharpness
Pb	Lead	Up	Photographic unsharpness
PET	Positron emission tomography	Us	Screen unsharpness
pH	Measure of acidity/alkalinity of a solution	Ut	Total unsharpness
		UV	Ultraviolet
PMS	Patient management system		
PQ	Phenidone hydroquinone	v	Object speed (velocity)
P s/n	Probability of positive response to noise	VDU	Visual display unit
P s/s	Probability of positive response to signal		
		W	Watt
Q	Hydroquinone	Y	Yttrium
QDE	Quantum detection efficiency		

Index

Abbreviations used: PACS, picture and archiving system.